NEW DEVELOPMENTS IN MEDICAL RESEARCH

NONEMERGENCY MEDICAL TRANSPORTATION: PROGRAM FEATURES AND ISSUES

NEW DEVELOPMENTS IN MEDICAL RESEARCH

Additional books in this series can be found on Nova's website under the Series tab.

Additional e-books in this series can be found on Nova's website under the e-book tab.

NEW DEVELOPMENTS IN MEDICAL RESEARCH

NONEMERGENCY MEDICAL TRANSPORTATION: PROGRAM FEATURES AND ISSUES

TREVOR DAVIS
EDITOR

New York

NOTICE TO THE READER

Library of Congress Cataloging-in-Publication Data

ISBN: 978-1-53610-118-8

Published by Nova Science Publishers, Inc. † New York

CONTENTS

PREFACE

Medicare and Medicaid provide nonemergency medical transportation (NEMT) services to eligible beneficiaries who need transportation to scheduled nonemergency care. The Centers for Medicare & Medicaid Services (CMS) administers Medicare NEMT benefits and is responsible for overseeing Medicaid at the federal level. Spending on NEMT under these programs was $2.7 billion in 2013—$1.2 billion for Medicare and $1.5 billion for Medicaid. Increased demand for NEMT because of increased Medicaid enrollment has led states to seek ways to more efficiently operate NEMT. This book examines key features of NEMT services under Medicare and Medicaid and how these services are delivered; steps CMS has taken to oversee NEMT under Medicare as well as Medicaid; and the challenges that exist in providing NEMT under Medicaid and steps that selected state Medicaid agencies have taken to address those challenges.

In: Nonemergency Medical Transportation ISBN: 978-1-53610-118-8
Editor: Trevor Davis

Chapter 1

NONEMERGENCY MEDICAL TRANSPORTATION: UPDATED MEDICAID GUIDANCE COULD HELP STATES*

United States Government Accountability Office

WHY GAO DID THIS STUDY

Medicare and Medicaid provide NEMT services to eligible beneficiaries who need transportation to scheduled nonemergency care. CMS administers Medicare NEMT benefits and is responsible for overseeing Medicaid at the federal level. Spending on NEMT under these programs was $2.7 billion in 2013—$1.2 billion for Medicare and $1.5 billion for Medicaid. Increased demand for NEMT because of increased Medicaid enrollment has led states to seek ways to more efficiently operate NEMT.

GAO was asked to review NEMT under Medicare and Medicaid. This report examines 1) key features of NEMT services under Medicare and Medicaid and how these services are delivered; 2) steps CMS has taken to oversee NEMT under Medicare as well as Medicaid; and 3) the challenges that exist in providing NEMT under Medicaid and steps that selected state Medicaid agencies have taken to address those challenges.

* This is an edited, reformatted and augmented version of a United States Government Accountability Office, Publication No. GAO-16-238, dated February 2016.

GAO reviewed key documents and interviewed officials from CMS; 15 selected states that range in terms of Medicaid enrollment and geography; and stakeholders, including transportation brokers, health plans, and health care and transportation industry groups.

What GAO Recommends

GAO recommends that the Secretary of HHS direct CMS to assess current Medicaid NEMT guidance and update it as needed. HHS concurred with our recommendation and provided technical comments which we incorporated as appropriate.

What GAO Found

The nonemergency medical transportation (NEMT) benefits offered by Medicare and Medicaid differ. Medicare provides NEMT via ambulance only when other means of transportation, such as a taxi or wheelchair van, would jeopardize the health of the beneficiary. Medicaid NEMT is generally available for beneficiaries who have no other means of transportation to medical services. States are responsible for the daily operations of their Medicaid programs and have discretion in how they deliver NEMT. Officials from 15 selected states reported using a variety of models to administer NEMT, including transportation brokers, which are entities that contract with states to administer NEMT services.

The Centers for Medicare & Medicaid Services (CMS), within the Department of Health and Human Services (HHS), oversees Medicare and Medicaid at the federal level, but this oversight varies by program. CMS generally uses regular program integrity activities—such as claims reviews—to oversee Medicare NEMT. Under Medicaid, CMS also uses regular oversight activities, and these include overseeing states' program integrity activities and periodically issuing guidance. However, some of CMS's guidance is outdated or may be of limited use because of legislative and other changes that affect Medicaid and states' NEMT programs. For example, a 1998 guidebook on NEMT contains outdated information on implementing NEMT transportation broker programs. Other more recent guidance is targeted for patients and providers rather than state Medicaid programs. However, these programs also benefit from updated guidance on strategies to ensure compliance with federal requirements while incorporating current practices to meet beneficiaries' needs. Guidance for state Medicaid programs is particularly important because NEMT is at high risk for fraud and abuse; some selected states and stakeholders GAO interviewed reported that updated guidance could be helpful. *Standards for Internal Control in the Federal Government* states that management should ensure adequate means of communicating with stakeholders. Effective communications can take many forms, including guidance. CMS officials reported that the agency is considering assessing whether additional NEMT guidance is needed, but has not set time frames for conducting this assessment.

GAO identified four types of challenges related to Medicaid NEMT and several steps taken by states to address some of these challenges. Challenges reported related to containing costs, maintaining program integrity, contracting with and overseeing vendors, and accessing NEMT. For example, states reported challenges containing NEMT costs due to increased NEMT utilization and reported implementing practices to help address these challenges. Such practices include setting fixed provider reimbursement fees that remained relatively constant in recent years. Officials from 7 of the 15 selected states and 6 stakeholders GAO interviewed reported that having information on how states administer NEMT and ways to address challenges could be helpful to states. Some of this information is available; for example, CMS reported collecting information on states' approaches through state Medicaid plans and posting this information on CMS's website. Other organizations, such as the Transit Cooperative Research Program, have or are in the process of collecting such information.

ABBREVIATIONS

CMS	Centers for Medicare & Medicaid Services
ESRD	end-stage renal disease
HHS	Department of Health and Human Services
MedPAC	Medicare Payment Advisory Commission
NEMT	nonemergency medical transportation
OIG	Office of Inspector General
PPACA	Patient Protection and Affordable Care Act
TCRP	Transit Cooperative Research Program

February 2, 2016

The Honorable Orrin G. Hatch
Chairman
The Honorable Ron Wyden
Ranking Member
Committee on Finance
United States Senate

The Honorable Johnny Isakson
United States Senate

Transportation to medical care is essential for many Medicare and Medicaid beneficiaries. A number of federal programs, including Medicare and Medicaid, can provide funding for nonemergency medical transportation (NEMT) service.[1] The Centers for Medicare & Medicaid Services (CMS), within the Department of Health and Human Services (HHS), administers the Medicare program, including NEMT benefits. CMS also oversees the design and operation of state Medicaid programs and their administration of NEMT benefits, but the states are responsible for the day-to-day operations of their Medicaid programs, including NEMT benefits. While NEMT is an important benefit for some beneficiaries, NEMT expenditures are relatively small compared to overall Medicare and Medicaid spending.[2] In calendar year 2013, spending on NEMT under these programs exceeded $2.7 billion—$1.2 billion and $1.5 billion for Medicare and Medicaid, respectively.[3] Medicare spending on NEMT has remained relatively stable, but Medicaid spending on NEMT has been steadily increasing since 2010, when it was 1 billion.[4] In an environment where Medicaid enrollment and spending on transportation are increasing, states are continually looking for more efficient ways to deliver trips to beneficiaries who need them, while at the same time maintaining program integrity.

You asked that we review NEMT services under Medicare and Medicaid. This report examines 1) key features of NEMT services under Medicare and Medicaid and how these services are administered; 2) steps CMS has taken to oversee NEMT under Medicare as well as Medicaid; and 3) the challenges that exist in providing NEMT under Medicaid, and steps that selected state Medicaid agencies have taken to address those challenges.

To identify key features of NEMT under Medicare and Medicaid, we reviewed applicable laws, regulations, and CMS guidance. To collect information on how NEMT is provided under Medicare, we interviewed CMS officials and stakeholders, including two patient advocacy organizations and one transportation industry group that are involved in coordinating transportation and reviewed reports by the Medicare Payment Advisory Commission (MedPAC) and HHS's Office of Inspector General (OIG).[5] To determine how NEMT is provided under Medicaid, the challenges faced by state Medicaid agencies, and steps that state Medicaid agencies and CMS are taking to address challenges, we reviewed HHS-OIG, state auditor, and Transit Cooperative Research Program (TCRP) reports.[6] We also reviewed other documents, such as state contracts and utilization and spending data, which were provided to us during interviews with officials from 15 state Medicaid agencies.[7] Additionally, we interviewed stakeholders, such as health care associations involved in Medicaid managed care, patient advocates, and a transportation industry group. We also visited 2 of the 15 selected states to obtain more in-depth information about challenges in providing NEMT, and interviewed officials with three health plans and two transportation brokers involved in providing NEMT.[8] Appendix I contains a more detailed discussion of our objectives, scope, and methodology.

We conducted this performance audit from January 2015 to January 2016 in accordance with generally accepted government auditing standards. Those standards require that we plan and perform the audit to obtain sufficient, appropriate evidence to provide a reasonable basis for our findings and conclusions based on our audit objectives. We believe that the evidence obtained provides a reasonable basis for our findings and conclusions based on our audit objectives.

BACKGROUND

Medicare and Medicaid are the federal government's two largest healthcare programs as measured by expenditures.

- Medicare is a healthcare insurance program for seniors, certain individuals with disabilities, and those with end-stage renal disease (ESRD), with Medicare expenditures totaling $613.3 billion for 53.8 million beneficiaries in 2014.[9] Under federal law, Medicare insurance includes hospital, medical, and prescription drug coverage. CMS administers the program, including safeguarding the program from loss due to fraud, waste, and abuse. Medicare is paid for through two trust funds held by the U.S. Treasury.[10]

- Medicaid is a joint federal-state health-financing program for low-income and medically needy individuals.[11] For 2014, estimated Medicaid spending totaled $499 billion for more than 65 million beneficiaries.[12] Medicaid operates within broad federal parameters, with states having flexibility in how they operate their programs and with CMS overseeing the design and operation of states' Medicaid programs. Medicaid is jointly financed by the federal government and the states, with the federal government matching most state Medicaid expenditures using a statutory formula—the Federal Medical Assistance Percentage rate—generally based on each state's per capita income relative to the national average.

Medicare and Medicaid, and their NEMT programs, are provided under both fee-for-service and managed care payment systems:

- Under fee-for-service, either CMS (for Medicare) or the state Medicaid agency enrolls NEMT providers.[13] Providers are paid on a per-service basis.[14]
- Under managed care, either CMS (for Medicare) or the state Medicaid agency contracts with health plans to provide covered health care services—which can include NEMT—in return for a fixed monthly payment per enrollee. Under Medicare managed care, private organizations offer health plans through the Medicare Advantage program.

GAO has designated both the Medicare and Medicaid programs as high risk because of concerns about the Medicare program's size, complexity, and susceptibility to mismanagement and improper payments, and because of our concerns about inadequate federal oversight over state Medicaid programs.[15] We have also reported concerns about program integrity in Medicaid managed care, specifically with regard to vulnerabilities in protecting against improper payments.[16]

Modes of Transportation, Program Eligibility, and other Key NEMT Features Are Different under Medicare and Medicaid

Although Medicare and Medicaid both offer NEMT services to their beneficiaries, based on the individual program requirements, certain key features of NEMT operate differently under the two programs, as described below (see table 1). These differences reflect fundamental differences between the two programs, Medicare being a healthcare insurance program administered at the federal level and Medicaid being a joint federal-state health financing program.

Medicare Key Features

Under Medicare, NEMT services are allowed to be delivered via ambulance transport to scheduled nonemergency medical services for some beneficiaries. For example, Medicare NEMT may cover ambulance transportation for a beneficiary with ESRD for scheduled, repeated, and nonemergency transports to and from dialysis treatments, if transportation by ambulance is medically necessary. Similarly, Medicare may cover ambulance transportation upon discharge from an inpatient hospital for transport to a skilled nursing facility or to a beneficiary's home, when medically necessary. The beneficiary must have a written order from a doctor stating that ambulance transportation is necessary due to the beneficiary's medical condition, and the trip must be to or from the nearest medical facility. Ambulance providers may be compensated on a fee-for-service basis or under a managed care arrangement.

Medicaid Key Features

Under Medicaid, states must ensure NEMT for beneficiaries who have no other means of transportation to needed medical services—such as doctors' appointments and various types of therapies—and can provide NEMT in a variety of ways. States have discretion, consistent with federal requirements, in how they deliver NEMT, including the mode of transportation used and the model used to provide NEMT.[17] For instance, state Medicaid officials we interviewed reported covering a variety of modes of transportation for NEMT trips, including buses, taxi cabs, and vans. States also reported paying beneficiaries and their family members or friends' mileage for using their personal vehicles to provide transportation to needed medical care.[18] While the modes of transportation used for NEMT across states were similar, state officials reported using a variety of models to administer NEMT, including paying for NEMT on a fee-for-service basis; contracting with managed care health plans to provide health care services, including NEMT, for a per-member, per-month fee; and contracting with transportation brokers to manage all or some aspects of NEMT on states' behalf.[19] Further, some of our 15 selected states use a mix of models for administering NEMT. See table 2 for examples of states' models for administering NEMT.

Table 1. Key Features of Nonemergency Medical Transportation (NEMT) under Medicare and Medicaid

	Medicare	Medicaid
Modes of transportation	Medicare beneficiaries receive ground ambulance transport services, which may include Basic Life Support, Advanced Life Support, or Specialty Care Transport.a	States may use a variety of modes including ambulances, wheelchair and standard vans, taxiand limousines, public transportation, volunteer drivers, and personal vehicles.b
Program eligibility	Medicare beneficiaries are eligible for NEMT when their medical condition at the time of transport for medical services is such that other means of transportation—such as a taxi, private car, wheelchair van, or other type of vehicle—would jeopardize his or her health.c	NEMT services are typically available to Medicaid beneficiaries when they have no other source of transportation to medical services.
Enrolling providers	Medicare Administrative Contractors enroll NEMT ambulance providers and Medicare Advantage Plans contract with ambulance providers to deliver NEMT.d	Each state determines its process and requirements for enrolling and verifying the credentials of NEMT providers.

Source: GAO analysis of information from CMS, HHS-OIG, and GAO reports. | GAO-16-238

[a]Basic Life Support services include basic, noninvasive interventions, such as administering oxygen. Advanced Life Support services involve invasive or specialty care, such as administering drugs intravenously. Specialty Care Transport involves ongoing care furnished by one or more professionals in an appropriate specialty, such as respiratory or cardiovascular care.

[b]States may pay beneficiaries and their family members or others mileage reimbursement for using private vehicles for trips to covered medical care when NEMT is claimed as an administrative expense and mileage reimbursement may also be available when, for example, reimbursement is issued by a vendor, such as a broker.

[c]Individuals enrolled in Medicare may also qualify for Medicaid, assuming they meet Medicaid eligibility requirements.

[d]Medicare Advantage Plans are a private health plan alternative to traditional Medicare.

Table 2. Examples of Selected State Models for Administering Medicaid Nonemergency Medical Transportation (NEMT)

Model	Description
Fee-for-service	States may pay NEMT providers a fee for each trip. States may choose to handle their fee-for-service system centrally or delegate responsibility to local officials. For example: •Wyoming officials reported paying NEMT providers a fee for each trip provided to eligible beneficiaries. •Colorado officials reported delegating responsibility for NEMT to county-level authorities. Under this arrangement, counties pay providers for each trip and then submit claims to the state for reimbursement.
Managed care	States may contract with health plans to provide health care services, which can include NEMT, to beneficiaries for a set per-member, per-month fee. Under these arrangements the state delegates all NEMT responsibilities, including developing a provider network, providing services, and paying for services, to the health plan. In turn, the health plan may choose to subcontract with a transportation broker to administer NEMT for their members. For example: •Tennessee officials reported contracting with health plans to provide NEMT to beneficiaries, and contracts require health plans to subcontract with transportation brokers to administer NEMT. •Officials from Illinois reported contracting with health plans to provide NEMT to beneficiaries, and health plans use a variety of methods to manage the NEMT benefit, such as managing the benefit in-house or subcontracting with a broker.
Transportation broker	Some states contract with transportation brokers to provide NEMT for beneficiaries who are not in managed care. States' contracts with brokers vary in terms of payment, broker responsibilities, service areas, and populations covered. For example: •Georgia officials reported contracting with five brokers for a per-member, per-month fee to administerall aspects of NEMT, including developing the NEMT provider network, fielding beneficiary calls, making trip arrangements, and paying providers. •New York officials reported contracting with six regional brokers to perform overall fee-for-service NEMT management—including operating a call center and making trip arrangements—for a per-Medicaid enrollee, per-month fee. The state maintains responsibility for other tasks, such as enrollingand paying NEMT providers. •Michigan officials reported contracting with a broker to administer NEMT for beneficiaries residing in the Detroit area and who are not enrolled in a managed care health plan.
Mixed model	States may choose to use more than one model to administer NEMT across their states. For example: •Arizona officials reported contracting with managed care health plans to provide NEMT to their members for a capitated fee and also paying for NEMT on a fee-for-service basis for beneficiarieswho are not enrolled in managed care health plans.

Source: Analysis of interviews conducted from May through June 2015 with officials from Medicaid agencies in 15 selected states. | GAO-16-238.

CMS Oversight of NEMT Varies by Program, with CMS Using a Range of Activities to Oversee Medicaid NEMT

CMS oversight of NEMT under Medicare and Medicaid varies. CMS oversees Medicare NEMT using its regular oversights activities—such as claim reviews. Under Medicaid, CMS uses a range of regular oversight activities to oversee states' operations of their NEMT programs, including reviewing and approving state Medicaid plans and amendments; issuing guidance; conducting a range of program integrity activities, such as claims and state program integrity reviews; and offering technical assistance upon request. While CMS periodically issues NEMT guidance, some of this guidance is outdated or may be otherwise limited.

CMS Uses Regular Oversight Activities to Monitor NEMT

Medicare NEMT

CMS oversees Medicare NEMT through CMS's regular program integrity activities. These include conducting pre- and post-payment claim reviews by Medicare Administrative Contractors and calculating the Medicare improper payment rate through the Comprehensive Error Rate Testing program.[20] CMS initiated a 3-year Medicare prior authorization demonstration program in December 2014. This program is intended to help reduce improper payments for NEMT services. The program requires prior authorization of scheduled, repetitive nonemergency ambulance transports to test whether prior authorization helps reduce expenditures while maintaining or improving quality of care.[21] New Jersey, Pennsylvania, and South Carolina were selected to initially implement this program because of their high utilization of nonemergency ambulance transports under Medicare and improper payment rates.[22] Subsequently, CMS plans to expand the demonstration program to include Delaware, the District of Columbia, Maryland, North Carolina, West Virginia, and Virginia on January 1, 2016, as required by the Medicare Access and CHIP Reauthorization Act of 2015 and plans to expand the program to all states beginning January 1, 2017, if the Secretary of HHS and Chief Actuary determine certain conditions will occur under the expansion.[23]

Medicaid NEMT

Under Medicaid, states are responsible for the daily oversight of their NEMT programs and CMS oversees states' operations using a range of regular oversight activities. Within broad federal parameters, states determine their own processes for overseeing their Medicaid NEMT programs, including verifying beneficiary eligibility, establishing provider requirements, and preventing improper payments. To oversee states' operations of their NEMT programs, CMS conducts a range of oversight activities, including:

- CMS reviews and approves Medicaid plans and state plan amendments, which outline how states administer their Medicaid programs, including their NEMT programs.[24]
- CMS periodically issues guidance on NEMT requirements. CMS has issued several pieces of guidance, including a guidebook, letters to state Medicaid Directors, and a toolkit, on different aspects of NEMT.
- CMS conducts a range of program integrity activities. First, CMS calculates a national-level improper payment error rate through the Payment Error Rate Measurement program. Second, CMS also contracts with entities to, among other things, audit claims, identify overpayments, and educate providers and others on Medicaid program integrity issues.[25] Third, CMS conducts state program integrity reviews. For example, CMS conducts program integrity reviews of state Medicaid agencies—which are done to identify vulnerabilities in state operations that warrant improvements or corrections—and has provided assistance to states to address those vulnerabilities. Agency officials reported that these reviews have included an assessment of states' oversight of NEMT providers since fiscal year 2011. Further, CMS's ongoing program integrity reviews in three states include an assessment of risks and vulnerabilities in NEMT services.[26] CMS also conducts special audits and investigations of traditionally high-risk areas, including NEMT. For example, CMS reported collaborating with one state, New York, to conduct a special investigation of the state's NEMT program.[27]
- CMS provides technical assistance and clarifying guidance upon request. For example, officials from one selected state reported working with CMS to identify options for redesigning their NEMT program that would be consistent with regulations.

CMS Issues Guidance on Medicaid NEMT, but Some Guidance Is Outdated or May Be Otherwise Limited

Although CMS periodically issues NEMT guidance, some guidance is outdated or may be otherwise limited because legislative and other changes have affected Medicaid and states' NEMT programs. For example:

- CMS issued a guidebook in 1998 on designing and operating a cost-effective Medicaid NEMT program. This guidebook included information on factors and challenges that could be considered when designing and operating an NEMT program—describing the advantages and disadvantages of providing NEMT under a brokerage system, operating NEMT in a managed care environment, and strategies to identify and prevent NEMT fraud and abuse—and suggestions to address these concerns.[28] However, this guidebook contains outdated information. For example, the guidebook describes limited cases when state Medicaid programs can use brokerages. However, the Deficit Reduction Act of 2005 changed the conditions under which states could use NEMT brokerages, which expanded the number of states that utilize NEMT brokers. The guidebook does not address these conditions as discussed further below.
- After the Deficit Reduction Act of 2005 was passed, CMS issued a letter to State Medicaid Directors in 2006 describing changes in the law, and final rules in 2009 for establishing NEMT brokerage programs under states Medicaid plans.[29] However, CMS has not assessed NEMT guidance to determine if updates are needed in light of recent changes. For example, since 2009, there have been changes to the Medicaid program such as expanding Medicaid as allowed under the Patient Protection and Affordable Care Act (PPACA), and states have made changes to their Medicaid programs.[30] These changes have increased Medicaid enrollment in some states resulting in more NEMT trips.
- More recently, CMS issued a NEMT program integrity tool kit in June 2014.[31] This toolkit includes educational materials summarizing the general scope of Medicaid-covered NEMT and key principles applicable to such coverage, such as trip eligibility and NEMT fraud and abuse definitions. However, these materials are targeted for patients and providers rather than state Medicaid programs. However, state Medicaid programs may also benefit from updated information

on strategies to implement a program integrity program that could help to prevent NEMT fraud and abuse.

Updated guidance is important because it is a way to communicate an entity's objectives to help ensure its objectives are carried out. State Medicaid agencies rely on it when designing and administering their NEMT programs to help ensure compliance with federal requirements while incorporating current practices to meet beneficiaries' needs. According to CMS officials, some states do not always understand the NEMT benefit, in part, because NEMT guidance is not specific to the benefit. For example, states must generally follow overarching federal Medicaid requirements in providing NEMT under their state plans, such as requirements on granting beneficiaries the freedom to choose to obtain Medicaid services from any provider that is qualified and willing to provide services, unless states establish an NEMT transportation brokerage program.[32] Officials from two states reported that clarifying NEMT requirements would be helpful and three stakeholders (one transportation broker and two industry groups) reported that additional NEMT guidance would be helpful. For example, a transportation broker reported that additional guidance would help prevent states from implementing unnecessarily stringent requirements, which could restrict the supply of providers and limit access to NEMT. *Standards for Internal Control in the Federal Government* states that management should ensure that there are adequate means of communicating with, and obtaining information from, external stakeholders that may have a significant impact on the agency's ability to achieve its goals.[33] Effective communication can take many forms such as through guidance, training, or publication of best practices. CMS officials reported that the agency is considering assessing whether additional NEMT guidance is needed, but has not established time frames for doing so.

Selected States Have Taken Steps to Address Some Medicaid NEMT Challenges, and Information on State NEMT Practices Is Available

Through our work, we identified a range of challenges related to providing NEMT and steps taken by some states to address these challenges. Challenges and steps identified were related to

- containing costs,
- maintaining program integrity,
- contracting with and overseeing vendors, and
- accessing NEMT.

State officials reported that information on the approaches other states take for administering NEMT and strategies to address challenges could help them address ongoing challenges. CMS and other organizations, such as TCRP, have collected or are in the process of collecting such information.

Containing Costs

Officials from selected states and stakeholders reported challenges containing Medicaid NEMT costs due to increased utilization and certain trip factors. Officials from nine of our selected states reported that NEMT utilization increased from 2012 to 2014 and reported varying reasons for the increase in trips.[34] Reported reasons for increased NEMT utilization included:

- increased Medicaid enrollment caused by expanding Medicaid as allowed under the PPACA and by the economic downturn;
- program changes, such as covering NEMT to more types of health care services, such as dental or mental health care; and
- greater awareness of the benefit among beneficiaries.

Officials from nine states and three stakeholders (two counties and a transportation broker) reported that certain trip factors—such as traveling long distances, needing specialized vehicles, and reaching rural locations—made it difficult to contain costs. Further, officials from three states reported that these types of trips are sometimes more costly, because officials may negotiate higher provider reimbursement rates, thus making containing costs more difficult.

Officials from selected states reported implementing varying practices to contain NEMT costs, including using payment mechanisms, coordinating with stakeholders, and implementing policies.[35] See table 3 for examples of selected state practices that could address challenges containing NEMT costs.

Table 3. Examples of Selected State Practices That Could Address Challenges in Containing Nonemergency Medical Transportation (NEMT) Costs

State may use varying practices to lower NEMT costs, including using payment mechanisms, coordinating with stakeholders, and implementing policies. For example:
• Tennessee officials reported including NEMT in its capitated payment to health plans to control NEMT costs.
• Louisiana officials reported setting fixed provider reimbursement fees that have remained relatively constant in recent years.
• Connecticut officials reported that the state department of transportation provided their broker with information on public transportation options and pick-up locations so the broker could provide transportation at the lowest cost that met beneficiaries' needs.
• Wyoming officials reported working with beneficiaries undergoing certain types of treatment, such as chemotherapy and dialysis, to identify treatment centers closer to their homes.
• Georgia officials reported that the state's geographic access standard limits travel to see a physician to 30 miles in urban areas, such as Atlanta.

Source: GAO analysis of interviews conducted from May through June 2015 with officials from 15 selected states. | GAO-16-238.

Maintaining Program Integrity

Officials from CMS and selected states identified program integrity challenges related to improper payments for trips, including paid trips that did not meet program requirements.[36] According to CMS officials, state Medicaid officials reported that Medicaid claim reviews revealed that NEMT providers overbilled and documented trips poorly and that overpayments tended to occur more frequently in states that delegate NEMT responsibility to counties where officials may not be familiar with documentation requirements. Officials from six states also reported improper payments for NEMT, and three of these states attributed improper payments to challenges documenting trips. For example, in its Single Audit Act audit report for the year ending on June 30, 2015, the Louisiana Legislative Auditor identified payments totaling more than $850,000 for trips that did not meet established policies, including requirements for accurately documenting services.[37] Studies have also identified improper payments for Medicaid NEMT trips. For example, HHS-OIG conducted reviews of samples of Medicaid claims over a 1 or 2 year period from 2005 through 2011 in five states—California, Hawaii, Nebraska,

New York, and Texas—and found that some paid NEMT trips did not meet federal and state requirements. HHS-OIG subsequently recommended that collectively, these states should refund the federal government about $63 million.[38]

CMS and state auditor reports, officials from selected states, and stakeholders also identified other program integrity challenges that could make NEMT vulnerable for fraud, waste, and abuse, including:

- *Enrolling providers:* In annual summary reports of comprehensive program integrity reviews, CMS identified one state that did not require and collect key information needed for effective oversight, such as criminal conviction information from NEMT providers, making the state vulnerable to enrolling problem providers in its NEMT program.[39] Further, officials from six states cited challenges obtaining certain information on NEMT providers that could reduce program risks. For example, officials from one state reported they cannot access information on criminal convictions in other states, making it harder to conduct thorough background checks that could reduce program risks.
- *Program inefficiencies:* State auditors in six states identified problems with states' implementation of NEMT programs that could lead to program inefficiencies.[40] For example, in 2012 the Washington State Auditor identified program risks in the state's Medicaid NEMT program, such as that the Medicaid agency did not require brokers to maintain consistent trip data and that the agency lacked written policies and procedures to ensure clear management and consistent processes. As a result, the state's six brokers reported inconsistent practices, which could lead to overbilling for trips. To address identified program risks, the state auditor recommended that the state, among other things, improve oversight, monitoring, and data analysis.[41]
- *Verifying eligibility:* Officials from selected states reported several challenges verifying that trips fall within the scope of Medicaid-covered NEMT. First, officials from two states reported challenges verifying beneficiary eligibility for Medicaid or the need for NEMT services. For example, the Medicaid agency, broker, and county officials from one state reported challenges verifying Medicaid enrollment because the state updates its Medicaid enrollment database daily; thus, beneficiaries who were enrolled in Medicaid when trips

were requested may not be enrolled on the days trips were provided. Second, officials from another state reported that it had challenges verifying that the beneficiary did not have other means of transportation. Third, officials from seven states reported challenges verifying that NEMT trips were to needed medical services. For instance, officials from two states reported challenges verifying the purpose of NEMT trips to certain pharmacies, including Target and Walmart, which carry non-medical products, such as food and clothing, in addition to drugs and medical supplies. In these cases, it was hard to determine whether NEMT was used appropriately, particularly when beneficiaries requested multiple NEMT trips to the pharmacy to pick up prescriptions that could potentially have been picked-up in a single trip.

Officials from all selected states reported taking at least one step to address these NEMT program integrity challenges. See table 4 for examples of selected state practices that could address challenges to maintaining NEMT program integrity.

Contracting with and Overseeing Vendors

Officials from four states cited challenges contracting with and overseeing vendors, such as health plans and transportation brokers, and officials from two of these states reported that challenges arose during periods of transition. For example, officials from one state reported that in the first year of contracting with multiple brokers, challenges with one broker's compliance with contractual requirements arose because the broker underestimated the resources needed to administer NEMT. State officials explained that under their prior method for delivering NEMT, they did not have complete information on trip volume or mode, making it difficult to determine the appropriate level of resources needed when requesting and evaluating vendors' contract proposals. Further, these state officials reported challenges developing metrics to monitor all brokers' compliance with certain contract requirements. For instance, brokers are required to furnish NEMT for all eligible trip requests, but officials in one state reported that about 1 percent of eligible trips requested by Medicaid beneficiaries are not provided. Without collecting complete information on NEMT trips under the state's previous system, identifying a reasonable proportion of missed trips under the state's new system to assess compliance with contract requirements has been difficult.

Table 4. Examples of Selected State Practices That Could Address Challenges in Maintaining Nonemergency Medical Transportation (NEMT) Program Integrity

Step	Description of step
Reviewing claims	States review Medicaid claims for NEMT to monitor providers'billing patterns and toidentify potential fraud.a
Suspending NEMT providers	States or their contracted vendors can suspend NEMT providers from the Medicaid program for not meeting program requirements or fraudulent activities. For example: •A Georgia official reported that its brokers will suspend providers from the Medicaid program when providers and vehicles do not meet state credentialing criteria. •Arizona officials reported suspending providers from the Medicaid program for credible allegations of fraud.
Including program integrity contract provisions	States include contract provisions requiring vendors, including health plans and transportation brokers, to implement program integrity efforts to prevent improper payments for paid NEMT trips.For example, Colorado's contract with a transportation broker requires the broker to verify that beneficiaries are eligible for Medicaid prior to and the day of providing NEMT trips and outlines NEMT eligibility criteria. Further, officials from all three transportation brokers we interviewed reported implementing steps to meet such requirements. For example: •Officials from one broker reported that they verify Medicaid eligibility twice—when they receive a request for NEMT and the day before NEMT is provided. •Officials with another broker told us that they sometimes call physicians' offices to verify that the beneficiary has a scheduled medical appointment.
Updating and clarifying requirements	States update and clarify guidance on NEMT billing documentation requirements. For example, California officials reported updating their provider manual to clarify NEMT billing and documentation requirements, and holding trainings to notify providers of current policies.
Reviewing protocols	States review vendor screening tools and protocols. For example, Tennessee officials reported reviewing and approving brokers' call centers' screening tools intended to prevent trips that are outside Medicaid-covered NEMT.b

Source: GAO analysis of interviews conducted from May through June 2015 with officials from 15 selected states and stakeholders. | GAO-16-238

[a]Federal laws authorize both state and federal entities to protect Medicaid from fraud, waste, and abuse. See, e.g., 42 U.S.C. §§ 1396a(a)(69) and 1396u-6. To meet requirements, state program integrity activities may include pre- and post-payment claim reviews to ensure appropriateness of payments and identify potentially fraudulent providers for further investigation.

[b]Tennessee officials reported that the state includes NEMT services in its contracts with health plans and requires health plans to contract with transportation brokers to manage the NEMT benefit.

Officials from all selected states that contract with health plans or transportation brokers to provide NEMT reported conducting monitoring activities, such as performing annual audits and site visits, to address challenges with contracting and overseeing vendors. See table 5 for examples of selected state practices that could address challenges contracting with and overseeing vendors.

Table 5. Examples of Selected State Practices that Could Address Challenges in Contracting with and Overseeing Nonemergency Medical Transportation (NEMT) Vendors

Step	Description of step
Monitoring vendor compliance	States monitor vendors to ensure compliance with contract requirements.For example: •Tennessee officials reported monitoring brokers by conducting annual site visits and listening to some calls received by call-centers to ensure staff are screening callers appropriately.[a] •A District of Columbia official reported conducting random checks of its broker's NEMT documents, such as provider enrollment documents, to ensure it is maintaining appropriate records to comply with contract requirements.
Reviewing NEMT data	States require brokers and health plans to periodically submit NEMT data for review. For example: •Colorado's contract requires its broker to submit monthly reports that include data on the number of trips authorized and scheduled, number of trips denied, and number of no-shows. •Louisiana officials reported that health plans are required to submit data monthly on beneficiaries' grievances and actions taken to address them.
Taking actions to address identified issues	States take actions to address identified compliance issues. For example: •A Georgia official reported working with brokers to address compliance issues. •Louisiana officials reported asking one of its health plans to terminate its relationship with a particularbroker because of performance issues, and the health plan complied with this request.

Source: GAO analysis of interviews conducted from May through June 2015 with officials from 15 selected states. | GAO-16-238.

[a]Tennessee officials reported that the state includes NEMT services in its contracts with health plans and requires health plans to contract with transportation brokers to manage the NEMT benefit.

Accessing NEMT

State officials and stakeholders reported challenges ensuring access to NEMT when the demand for trips exceeded the supply of NEMT providers. Officials generally identified four factors that affected the supply of NEMT providers—geographic location, specialty providers, provider requirements, and beneficiary and provider no-shows. Specifically, officials from seven states and nine stakeholders reported a low supply of NEMT providers in rural areas, and officials from seven states and four stakeholders reported a low supply of specialty vehicles, such as stretcher or wheelchair vans. Officials from two states and three stakeholders reported that state transportation provider requirements may limit the number of or deter providers from entering the Medicaid provider pool. Lastly, officials from seven states and five stakeholders reported that beneficiaries or providers sometimes did not show-up or were late for trips, thus tying-up NEMT resources.

Officials from selected states reported taking steps to address access challenges, including broadening the provider networks and reviewing state provider requirements. See table 6 for examples of selected state practices that could address NEMT access challenges.

Information on Leading Practices

Officials from seven selected states and six stakeholders reported that having information on how other states administer NEMT and address challenges could help them address ongoing challenges. For example, officials from one state reported that they plan to make changes to the state's NEMT program to address ongoing challenges and that they have spoken to officials from other states to learn about how they administer NEMT. In spite of these efforts, officials from this state reported that they could not identify any state NEMT programs that could accommodate all beneficiaries well and that information on current leading practices for developing a robust NEMT program would be helpful. An official from another state reported that having information on leading practices would help to identify approaches for improving NEMT program integrity.

Table 6. Examples of Selected State Practices that Could Address Challenges in Accessing Nonemergency Medical Transportation (NEMT)

Step	Description of step
Broadening NEMT provider network	States increase the supply of NEMT providers by: •paying mileage reimbursement to beneficiaries and beneficiaries' family members or friends who use personal vehicles to drive to needed medical services;a •using volunteer drivers; and •coordinating with a variety of local organizations. For example, officials from a rural county in Colorado reported coordinating with a local casino that ran a van to ensure access to NEMT for a beneficiary.
Reviewing state provider requirements	States review their provider requirements to ensure they do not restrict the number of providers able to enroll in the Medicaid program. For example, Colorado officials reported plans to review state provider requirements and potentially work with the legislature to address requirements that affect the Medicaid provider supply.
Using probation periods or suspensions	States use probation periods or suspensions to address patterns of no-shows. For example, •Missouri officials reported that providers can be terminated from the broker's NEMT provider network after multiple no-shows; and •Tennessee officials reported that brokers subcontracting with TennCare health plans use a probationary period to handle beneficiary no-shows.b
Coordinating with health plans	States and brokers work with health plans to address beneficiary no-shows. For example, officials fromColorado's transportation broker reported working with beneficiaries' health plans when they receive repeated reports of beneficiaries not showing-up for NEMT.

Source: GAO analysis of interviews conducted from May through June 2015 with officials from 15 selected states and stakeholders. | GAO-16-238.

[a]According to the Centers for Medicare & Medicaid Services, states may pay beneficiaries and their family members or others mileage reimbursement for using their private vehicles for trips to covered medical care generally when NEMT is claimed as an administrative expense or when reimbursement is issued by vendor, such as a broker.

[b]TennCare is Tennessee's Medicaid program. State officials reported that the state includes NEMT services in its contracts with health plans and requires health plans to contract with transportation brokers to manage the NEMT benefit.

Some information on approaches for administering NEMT and leading practices is available. CMS reported that it collects information on state approaches for administering NEMT through state Medicaid plans and state plan amendments and maintains this information on Medicaid.gov.[42] Further, CMS collects information on Medicaid programs and noteworthy program integrity practices, including those related to NEMT, as part of its program integrity reviews. Other organizations have or are in the process of collecting information on states' approaches to administer their Medicaid NEMT programs. For example, TCRP is conducting a study evaluating the effects of different options for providing Medicaid NEMT on access and coordination. As part of this work, TCRP officials reported collecting information from all 50 states and the District of Columbia on their approaches for administering NEMT.

CONCLUSION

For some Medicaid beneficiaries, NEMT is a critical service to ensure that they are able to travel to medical appointments. Although a small proportion of total Medicaid spending, increases in the number of Medicaid beneficiaries and other factors have led to increased demand and spending on Medicaid NEMT. States take different approaches to administering Medicaid NEMT and rely on CMS guidance when designing their NEMT programs to ensure compliance with federal requirements. While CMS periodically issues guidance on NEMT, current guidance may be out of date or otherwise limited. For example, CMS issued a NEMT guidebook in 1998, but this guidebook does not include current guidance on implementing a transportation brokerage program under a state Medicaid plan. Some selected states and stakeholders told us that clarifying NEMT guidance would be helpful. As described in *Standards for Internal Control in the Federal Government*, management should ensure adequate means of communicating with, and obtaining information from, external stakeholders. CMS officials reported that the agency is considering assessing whether additional NEMT guidance is needed, but has not set any timeframes for conducting that assessment.

RECOMMENDATIONS

To ensure states have appropriate and current guidance to assist them in designing and administering Medicaid NEMT, we recommend the Secretary of HHS direct CMS to assess current Medicaid NEMT guidance and update that guidance as needed.

AGENCY COMMENTS

We provided a copy of the draft to HHS. HHS concurred with our recommendation and provided technical comments, which we incorporated as appropriate. HHS's comments are reprinted in appendix II.

Carolyn L. Yocom
Director
Health Care

Mark Goldstein
Director
Physical Infrastructure

APPENDIX I: OBJECTIVES, SCOPE, AND METHODOLOGY

This report addresses non-emergency medical transportation (NEMT) under Medicare and Medicaid and examines: 1) the key features of NEMT services under Medicare and Medicaid and how services are administered; 2) steps that the Centers for Medicare & Medicaid (CMS) have taken to oversee NEMT under Medicare as well as Medicaid; and 3) the challenges that exist in providing NEMT under Medicaid and steps that selected state Medicaid agencies have taken to address those challenges.

To determine the key features of NEMT under Medicare and Medicaid and how services are administered, as well as to determine steps that CMS has taken to oversee NEMT under Medicare and Medicaid, we reviewed applicable laws, regulations, and CMS guidance. We also reviewed key reports, such as Medicare Payment Advisory Commission, Department of Health and Human Services-Office of Inspector General (HHS-OIG), and

Transit Cooperative Research Program (TCRP) reports, and prior GAO reports.[1] Additionally, we conducted searches in bibliographic databases—including Medline, National Technical Information Service, WorldCat PAIS International, and Social Services Abstracts—to identify additional literature on NEMT under Medicare and Medicaid. We screened search results and identified studies for relevance to our research objectives and selected those that focused on delivery of NEMT services under Medicaid and Medicare. We interviewed CMS and HHS-OIG officials, as well as two patient advocates and a transportation industry group involved in coordinating transportation. In addition, for Medicaid, we interviewed officials from 15 selected state Medicaid agencies. We selected a non-probability sample of states based on a mix of considerations, including Medicaid enrollment and spending, the approaches states use to deliver NEMT, geographic distribution, and whether or not states have expanded Medicaid under the Patient Protection and Affordable Care Act (PPACA).[2] The selected states were: Arizona, California, Colorado, Connecticut, District of Columbia, Georgia, Illinois, Louisiana, Maine, Michigan, Missouri, New York, Ohio, Tennessee, Washington, and Wyoming.[3] We also reviewed documents from states, such as contracts with health plans and organizations providing NEMT, and utilization and spending data.

To determine the challenges that exist in providing NEMT and steps that state Medicaid agencies are taking, we screened and identified studies from the sources identified above, and selected and reviewed studies that focused on challenges in providing NEMT under Medicaid, as well as HHS-OIG and state auditor reports. We also interviewed CMS and HHSOIG officials, two patient advocates, and a transportation industry group that are involved in coordinating transportation, two healthcare industry associations that are knowledgeable about providing NEMT under Medicaid, including Medicaid managed care, and officials from the 15 selected state Medicaid agencies. In order to obtain more in-depth information about challenges, we visited two states—Louisiana and Colorado—to interview officials involved in providing NEMT. We selected these two states because they use more than one model to provide NEMT, including using at least one broker, and have both rural and urban populations. In Louisiana, we interviewed officials from two health plans that had contracts with the state for more than 1 year and serve more than 50 percent of the Medicaid beneficiaries enrolled in managed care, as well as the two transportation brokers that provide NEMT.[4] In Colorado, we interviewed the transportation broker Colorado uses for the Denver metropolitan area, a health care plan that serves Medicaid beneficiaries in

Colorado and officials in two counties outside of the Denver metropolitan area that are responsible for providing NEMT to their residents.

APPENDIX II: COMMENTS FROM THE DEPARTMENT OF HEALTH AND HUMAN SERVICES

DEPARTMENT OF HEALTH & HUMAN SERVICES   OFFICE OF THE SECRETARY

Assistant Secretary for Legislation
Washington, DC 20201

JAN 2 0 2016

Carolyn Yocom
Director, Health Care
U.S. Government Accountability Office
441 G Street NW
Washington, DC 20548

Dear Ms. Yocom:

Attached are comments on the U.S. Government Accountability Office's (GAO) report entitled, "*Nonemergency Medical Transportation: Updated Medical Guidance Could Help States*" (GAO-16-238).

The Department appreciates the opportunity to review this report prior to publication.

Sincerely,

Jim R. Esquea
Assistant Secretary for Legislation

Attachment

GENERAL COMMENTS OF THE DEPARTMENT OF HEALTH AND HUMAN SERVICES (HHS) ON THE GOVERNMENT ACCOUNTABILITY OFFICE'S DRAFT REPORT ENTITLED: NONEMERGENCY MEDICAL TRANSPORTAION: UPDATED MEDICAID GUIDANCE COULD HELP STATES (GAO-16-238)

The Department of Health and Human Services (HHS) appreciates the opportunity to review and comment on this draft report. HHS is strongly committed to eliminating fraud, waste, and abuse in the Medicare and Medicaid non-emergency medical transportation (NEMT) benefits and appropriately overseeing States in the administration of NEMT benefits.

Medicare beneficiaries are eligible for NEMT if such transportation is needed to obtain treatment or diagnose a health condition and the use of any other transportation method could endanger a beneficiary's health. For Medicaid, NEMT is an important benefit as it enables Medicaid beneficiaries with no other means of transportation to get to and from providers. Access to transportation can improve the medical outcomes of Medicaid beneficiaries and can help avoid costly ambulance trips or emergency room visits.

As mentioned in the GAO report, HHS uses different oversight strategies for NEMT benefits under Medicare and Medicaid to address the specific needs of each program. Under Medicare, HHS oversees NEMT through its regular program integrity activities, which include conducting pre- and post-payment claims reviews, determining a service-specific improper payment rate through the Comprehensive Error Rate Testing program, and operating a prior authorization program for repetitive, scheduled non-emergent ambulance transport in select states. Under Medicaid, HHS oversees states' operations of NEMT programs in a variety of ways, including review and approval of Medicaid State plans and amendments, claims review, technical assistance, and issuance of guidance materials.

For Medicaid, HHS provides technical assistance to states as they implement and improve their NEMT program. This technical assistance enables states to make informed decisions on their program goals and objectives. It is used by states during the state plan review process and on an ad hoc basis depending upon the state's unique needs. In June 2014, HHS issued an NEMT program integrity toolkit to educate patients and providers about the scope of the Medicaid NEMT benefit. The toolkit also identifies common NEMT fraud and abuse issues and helps beneficiaries report potential fraud and abuse. These materials were updated in September 2015 and can be accessed online.[1]

For Medicare NEMT benefits, HHS launched a prior authorization model for Medicare-covered repetitive, scheduled non-emergent ambulance transports in South Carolina, New Jersey, and Pennsylvania in December 2014. In accordance with requirements in the Medicare Access and CHIP Reauthorization Act of 2015, in January 2016, CMS expanded this model to Delaware, the District of Columbia, Maryland, North Carolina, Virginia, and West Virginia and will evaluate whether to expand the model nationwide. CMS is testing whether prior authorization helps reduce expenditures while maintaining or improving quality of care. CMS believes using a prior authorization process will help make sure services are provided in compliance with Medicare coverage, coding, and payment rules before services are rendered and claims are paid.

[1] https://www.cms.gov/medicare-medicaid-coordination/fraud-prevention/medicaid-integrity-education/downloads/nemt-booklet.pdf

GENERAL COMMENTS OF THE DEPARTMENT OF HEALTH AND HUMAN SERVICES (HHS) ON THE GOVERNMENT ACCOUNTABILITY OFFICE'S DRAFT REPORT ENTITLED: NONEMERGENCY MEDICAL TRANSPORTAION: UPDATED MEDICAID GUIDANCE COULD HELP STATES (GAO-16-238)

GAO's recommendations and HHS' responses are below.

GAO Recommendation
To ensure states have appropriate and current guidance to assist them in designing and administering Medicaid NEMT, we recommend the Secretary of HHS direct CMS to assess current Medicaid NEMT guidance and update that guidance as needed.

HHS Response
HHS concurs with GAO's recommendation. HHS will examine current Medicaid NEMT guidance and publish or update additional guidance as necessary to assist states in designing and administering the Medicaid NEMT benefit.

HHS thanks GAO for their efforts on this issue and looks forward to working with GAO on this and other issues in the future.

End Notes

[1] We found that 42 programs across six federal departments—Agriculture, Education, Health and Human Services, Housing and Urban Development, Transportation, and Veterans Affairs—can provide funding for NEMT. See GAO, *Transportation Disadvantaged Populations: Nonemergency Medical Transportation Not Well Coordinated, and Additional Federal Leadership Needed*, GAO-15-110 (Washington, D.C.: Dec. 10, 2014).

[2] According to CMS's National Health Expenditure Data, Medicare and Medicaid expenditures in 2013 totaled more than one trillion dollars—about $586 billion for Medicare and $449 billion for Medicaid.

[3] We used Medicare NEMT paid claims data from the Part B National Summary Data File for calendar year 2013. Although this data does not include NEMT spending under Medicare Part A, CMS officials indicated that NEMT rarely occurs under Medicare Part A. Total Medicaid spending for NEMT is incomplete. States have the option to report NEMT as a medical assistance expense or an administrative expense. The amount reported includes spending by those states that have selected to report NEMT as a medical assistance expense, but does not include spending by states that chose to report NEMT as an administrative expense.

[4] Medicare Part B spending on NEMT was $1.24 billion in 2010, $1.26 billion in 2011, and $1.24 billion in 2012. Medicaid spending on NEMT was $1.01 billion in 2010, $1.15 billion in 2011, and $1.41 billion in 2012.

[5] MedPAC is an independent congressional agency established by the Balanced Budget Act of 1997 (Public Law 105-33) to advise the U.S. Congress on issues affecting the Medicare program.

[6] TCRP is a cooperative effort between public and private entities, such as the Federal Transit Administration and the Transportation Research Board, which conducts research and provides information on transportation issues.

[7] We selected a non-probability sample of state Medicaid agencies based on a variety of considerations, including Medicaid enrollment, Medicaid spending, methods of delivering NEMT, and geographic diversity. Selected states include: Arizona, California, Colorado, Connecticut, District of Columbia, Georgia, Illinois, Louisiana, Maine, Michigan, Missouri, New York, Ohio, Tennessee, Washington, and Wyoming. Ohio did not respond to our inquiry. Results of our interviews are not generalizable.

[8] We also visited Colorado and Louisiana. We selected these two states because they use more than one model to provide NEMT, including using at least one broker, and have both rural and urban populations. While in those states, we interviewed the transportation brokers involved in providing NEMT. States may contract with transportation brokers to administer NEMT services. In general, brokers can be public or private individuals or entities. While in Colorado, we also interviewed officials from two counties that were responsible for providing NEMT.

[9] See The Boards of Trustees, *2015 Annual Report of the Boards of Trustees of the Federal Hospital Insurance and Federal Supplementary Medical Insurance Trust Funds* (Washington, D.C.: July 22, 2015).

[10] The Social Security Act established the Federal Hospital Insurance and Supplementary Medical Insurance Trust Funds. These trust funds can generally only be used to cover the costs to operate and administer the Medicare program. The Federal Hospital Insurance Trust Fund is financed primarily by payroll taxes, income from interest earnings on Treasury securities, and a portion of income taxes collected on Social Security benefits. The Federal Supplementary Medical Insurance Trust Fund is financed primarily by monthly beneficiary premiums, income from the General Fund of the Treasury, and interest earnings on Treasury securities. See 42 U.S.C. §§ 1395 and 1395t.

[11] Individuals enrolled in Medicare may also qualify for Medicaid services, assuming they meet Medicaid income and asset requirements. These individuals are considered to be dually eligible for Medicare and Medicaid.

[12] Centers for Medicare & Medicaid Services, Office of the Actuary, 2014 Actuarial Report on the Financial Outlook for Medicaid (Baltimore, MD: 2013).

[13] Medicare providers are enrolled through contractors, known as Medicare Administrative Contractors. We discuss Medicare Administrative Contractors in more detail later in the report.

[14] CMS distinguishes between providers that are based in an institution, such as a hospital, and suppliers that are not based at an institution, such as a local fire department, public emergency medical services agency, or private for-profit company. For purposes of this report, we use the term "providers" when referring to all providers and suppliers.

[15] See GAO, *High-Risk Series: An Update,* GAO-15-290 (Washington, D.C: Feb. 11, 2015).

[16] See GAO, *Medicaid Program Integrity: Increased Oversight Needed to Ensure Integrity of Growing Managed Care Expenditures,* GAO-14-341 (Washington, D.C., May 19, 2014).

[17] Medicaid's NEMT regulation requires state Medicaid plans to ensure necessary transportation for beneficiaries to and from providers. See 42 C.F.R. § 431.53. These plans are agreements between a state and the federal government that describe how states will administer their Medicaid programs. States may choose to amend their Medicaid policies and operations described in their state plan using a state plan amendment. CMS reviews and approves state Medicaid plans and state plan amendments. While states may not exclude coverage of mandatory benefits such as NEMT under their state plans, they may place appropriate limits on a service based on such criteria as medical necessity or on utilization control procedures, see 42 C.F.R. § 440.230(d), or they may seek a waiver of the NEMT requirement in

connection with a Medicaid demonstration project under section 1115 of the Social Security Act, see 42 U.S.C. § 1315(a). This provision authorizes the Secretary of HHS to waive certain federal Medicaid requirements for experimental, pilot, or demonstration projects that, in the Secretary's judgment, are likely to assist in promoting Medicaid objectives.

[18] States may pay beneficiaries and their family members or friends mileage reimbursement for using their private vehicles to provide transportation to needed medical care if the state provides NEMT as an administrative expense. Brokers that provide NEMT for states may also reimburse mileage for beneficiaries who use their personal vehicles.

[19] The Deficit Reduction Act of 2005 provided authorization for states to enter into agreements with transportation brokers to administer Medicaid NEMT under their state plans. In general, transportation brokers can be public or private entities and must be selected through a competitive bidding process. Pub. L. No. 109-171, § 6083, 120 Stat. 4, 120-121 (Feb. 8, 2006) and implementing regulations at 42 C.F.R. § 440.170(a)(4).

[20] The Comprehensive Error Rate Testing program is used to calculate the Medicare feefor-service improper payment rate and pre- and post-payment claim reviews by Medicare contractors.

[21] A repetitive ambulance service is defined as medically necessary ambulance transportation that is furnished for three or more round-trips during a 10-day period; or at least one round-trip per week for at least 3 weeks. The Middle Class Tax Relief and Job Creation Act of 2012 directed MedPAC to study payments to ambulance providers and submit a report to Congress by June 15, 2013. Specifically, the law directed the Commission to examine temporary add-on payments for ambulance providers, which at the time were scheduled to expire at the end of 2012. Pub. L. No. 112-96, § 3007(e), 126 Stat. 156, 190 (Feb. 22, 2012). In June 2013, MedPAC reported that claims for nonemergency ambulance trips per fee-for-service beneficiary increased 9.9 percent from 2007 to 2011, and that more pronounced growth had occurred in ambulance transports to and from dialysis facilities. MedPAC also found that six states had higher than average spending on nonemergency ambulance transport per dialysis beneficiary than other states. According to CMS officials, New Jersey, Pennsylvania, and South Carolina ranked in the top three in terms of total Medicare expenditures for NEMT. Medicare Payment Advisory Commission, *Report to the Congress: Medicare and the Health Care Delivery System* (Washington, D.C.: June 14, 2013), 167.

[22] Certain stakeholders have raised concerns that patients with ESRD in the demonstration states have experienced problems accessing NEMT under Medicare. CMS officials said that access to the Medicare transportation benefit is an issue for some Medicare beneficiaries. However, the officials noted that Medicare only allows transportation that is medically necessary to avoid jeopardizing the beneficiary's health. According to CMS officials, the agency has increased education to beneficiaries as well as to medical and transportation providers and suppliers and also intends to expand educational efforts as the demonstration program is expanded.

[23] The Secretary of Health and Human Services may expand the duration and the scope of the demonstration program if the Secretary determines that such an expansion is expected to reduce spending without reducing the quality of care or improve the quality of care without increasing spending, if the Chief Actuary certifies that such expansion would reduce (or would not result in any increase in) net program spending, and if the Secretary determines that such expansion would not deny or limit the coverage or provision of benefits for applicable individuals. Pub. L. No. 114-10, § 515(b), 129 Stat. 87, 174-175 (Apr. 16, 2015). See 42 U.S.C. §§ 1395m(l) and 1315a(c).

[24] CMS also reviews states' waiver applications. We discuss NEMT waivers in more detail in GAO, *Medicaid: Efforts to Exclude Nonemergency Transportation Not Widespread, but Raise Issues for Expanded Coverage,* GAO-16-221 (Washington, D.C.: Jan. 15, 2016).

[25] See 42 U.S.C. § 1396u-6(b).

[26] Officials reported conducting these program integrity reviews in Delaware, North Carolina, and Vermont and anticipated issuing results of these reviews in 2016.

[27] Officials anticipated that audit results will be available in 2016.

[28] See Health Care Financing Administration and the National Association of State Medicaid Directors' Non-Emergency Transportation Technical Advisory Group, *Designing and Operating Cost-Effective Medicaid Non-Emergency Transportation Programs A Guidebook for State Medicaid Agencies,* (Washington, D.C.: Aug. 1998).

[29] See Centers for Medicare & Medicaid Services, State Medicaid Director Letter, Mar. 31, 2006, SMDL #06-009, accessed Oct. 28, 2015, https://downloads.cms.gov/cmsgov/archived-downloads/SMDL/downloads/SMD06009.pdf; and 42 C.F.R. § 440.170.

[30] Pub. L. No. 111-148, 124 Stat. 119 (Mar. 23, 2010), as amended by the Health Care and Education Reconciliation Act of 2010, Pub. L. No. 111-152, 124 Stat. 1029 (Mar. 30, 2010). PPACA allows states to expand Medicaid to cover previously ineligible categories, such as childless adults with incomes at or below 138 percent of the federal poverty level. As of September 2015, 29 states and the District of Columbia have expanded Medicaid.

[31] This toolkit was updated in September, 2015, See Centers for Medicare & Medicaid Services, *Program Integrity: Non Emergency Medical Transportation Toolkit,* (2014: Baltimore, MD), accessed Nov. 11, 2015, https://www.cms.gov/Medicare-Medicaid-Coordination/Fraud-Prevention/Medicaid-Integrit y-Education/nemt.html.

[32] See 42 C.F.R. § 431.51.

[33] See GAO, *Standards for Internal Control in the Federal Government,* GAO/AIMD-00.21.3.1 (Washington, D.C.: Nov. 1999).

[34] Officials from 13 states provided us with data on NEMT utilization for 2012 and 2014.

[35] GAO previously reported that improved coordination can reduce transportation costs. See GAO-15-110.

[36] We did not estimate the amount of improper payments for NEMT. However, we previously reported that overall improper payments for Medicaid services are a significant cost to the federal government, with the federal share estimated at $17.5 billion in fiscal year 2014. See GAO-15-290. NEMT represents a small component of Medicaid spending.

[37] See Louisiana Legislative Auditor, *State of Louisiana Single Audit Report For the Year Ended June 30, 2014,* Report ID No. 80140112 (Baton Rouge, LA: Mar. 3, 2015). See 31 U.S.C Chapter 75 for the audit requirements under the Single Audit Act.

[38] We reviewed 10 reports by HHS-OIG on Medicaid NEMT that were published from 2010 through March 2015. See, for example, Department of Health and Human Services, Office of Inspector General, *California Claimed Medicaid Reimbursement for Some Nonemergency Medical Transportation Services That Did Not Comply with Federal And State Requirements*, A-09-13-02033 (Washington, D.C.: Jan. 2015); and Department of Health and Human Services, Office of Inspector General, *Texas Did Not Always Comply With Federal And State Requirements for Claims Submitted for the Nonemergency Medical Transportation Program*, A-06-12-00053 (Washington, D.C.: Oct. 2014).

[39] See Centers for Medicare & Medicaid Services, *Annual Summary Report of Comprehensive Program Integrity Reviews*, (Baltimore, MD: June 2012); and Centers for Medicare & Medicaid Services, *Annual Summary Report of Comprehensive Program Integrity Reviews*, (Baltimore, MD: June 2014). Federal law requires the Secretary of HHS to exclude

individuals convicted of certain crimes, such as convictions relating to patient neglect or abuse and felony convictions related to health care fraud, from participation in federal health care programs, including Medicaid, generally for a minimum of 5 years. Federal law authorizes the Secretary to exclude individuals convicted of other crimes, such as misdemeanor convictions relating to health care fraud, generally for a minimum of 3 years. See 42 U.S.C. § 1320a-7(a), (b)(1)-(3), (c)(3)(B), (D).

[40] We contacted state auditors in all 50 states and the District of Columbia and received reports from auditors in seven states: Florida, Maryland, Michigan, Missouri, Washington, West Virginia, and Wisconsin.

[41] See Washington State Auditor, *Non-Emergency Medical Transportation—Management Letter,* (Olympia, WA: June 14, 2012). In response to the state auditor's findings, Washington officials reported taking steps to address risks and protect NEMT program integrity.

[42] Information on approaches for administering NEMT may not be available for every state because state plan amendments approved prior to the existence of Medicaid.gov are not available on the website.

End Notes for Appendix I

[1] TCRP is a cooperative effort between public and private entities, such as the Federal Transit Administration and the Transportation Research Board, which conducts research and provides information on transportation issues.

[2] Pub. L. No. 111-148, 124 Stat. 119 (Mar. 23, 2010), as amended by the Health Care and Education Reconciliation Act of 2010, Pub. L. No. 111-152, 124 Stat. 1029 (Mar. 30, 2010).

[3] Ohio did not respond to our inquiry.

[4] States may contract with brokers to provide NEMT services for Medicaid beneficiaries to access medical care or services through a competitive bidding process. NEMT services may be provided under contract with public or private individuals or entities and transportation services can include, among other things, wheelchair vans, taxis, stretcher cars, or bus passes.

In: Nonemergency Medical Transportation
Editor: Trevor Davis
ISBN: 978-1-53610-118-8

Chapter 2

MEDICAID: EFFORTS TO EXCLUDE NONEMERGENCY TRANSPORTATION NOT WIDESPREAD, BUT RAISE ISSUES FOR EXPANDED COVERAGE*

United States Government Accountability Office

ABBREVIATIONS

CMS	Centers for Medicare & Medicaid Services
FPL	federal poverty level
HHS	Department of Health and Human Services
NEMT	nonemergency medical transportation
PPACA	Patient Protection and Affordable Care Act

WHY GAO DID THIS STUDY

Medicaid, a federal-state health financing program for certain low-income individuals, offers NEMT benefits to individuals who are unable to provide their own transportation to medical appointments. This benefit can be an

* This is an edited, reformatted and augmented version of The United States Government Accountability Office publication, GAO-16-221, dated January 2016.

important safety net for program enrollees as research has identified the lack of transportation as affecting Medicaid enrollees' access to services. Under PPACA, states can opt to expand eligibility for Medicaid to certain adults. However, some states have excluded the NEMT benefit for these newly eligible enrollees by obtaining a waiver of the requirement under the authority of a Medicaid demonstration project.

GAO was asked to explore state efforts to exclude the NEMT benefit for newly eligible Medicaid enrollees, and the potential implications of such efforts. This report examines (1) the extent to which states have excluded this benefit for newly eligible enrollees, and (2) the potential implications of such efforts on enrollees' access to services.

GAO contacted the 30 states that expanded Medicaid under PPACA as of September 30, 2015; reviewed relevant documents and interviewed officials in the 3 states that have taken efforts to exclude the NEMT benefit; reviewed prior research on transportation for disadvantaged populations; and interviewed officials from CMS, the federal agency that oversees Medicaid, and 10 research and advocacy groups based on referrals from subject-matter experts and knowledge of the NEMT benefit.

What GAO Found

States' efforts to exclude nonemergency medical transportation (NEMT) benefits from enrollees who are newly eligible for Medicaid under the Patient Protection and Affordable Care Act (PPACA) are not widespread. Of the 30 states that expanded Medicaid as of September 30, 2015, 25 reported that they did not undertake efforts to exclude the NEMT benefit for newly eligible enrollees, 3 states reported pursuing such efforts, and 2 states—New Jersey and Ohio—did not respond to GAO's inquiry. However, the Centers for Medicare & Medicaid Services (CMS), within the Department of Health and Human Services (HHS), indicated that neither New Jersey nor Ohio undertook efforts to exclude the NEMT benefit.

Two of the three states pursuing efforts to exclude the NEMT benefit—Indiana and Iowa—have received waivers from CMS to exclude the benefit, and are in different stages of evaluating the effect these waivers have on enrollees' access to care.

- Indiana's draft evaluation design describes plans to survey enrollee and provider experiences to assess any effect from excluding the NEMT benefit.
- Iowa's evaluation largely found comparable access between enrollees with and without the NEMT benefit; however, it also found that newly eligible enrollees beneath the federal poverty level tended to need more transportation assistance or have more unmet needs than those with higher incomes.
- Officials from the groups that GAO interviewed identified potential implications of excluding the NEMT benefit, such as a decrease in enrollee access to services and an increase in the costs of coverage. For example, nearly all of the groups indicated that excluding the NEMT benefit would impede access to services, particularly for those living in rural areas, as well as those with chronic health conditions.

* * *

January 15, 2016

The Honorable Ron Wyden
Ranking Member
Committee on Finance
United States Senate

The Honorable Frank Pallone, Jr.
Ranking Member
Committee on Energy and Commerce
House of Representatives

Recognizing the importance of transportation for many Americans' access to needed medical services, states are required to provide through their Medicaid programs—a federal-state health financing program for certain low-income and medically needy individuals—a nonemergency medical transportation (NEMT) benefit to individuals who are unable to provide their own transportation to medical appointments. A lack of transportation can be a barrier to accessing health care, particularly among low-income populations. For example, we previously reported that Medicaid enrollees most commonly cited a lack of transportation as the reason for delaying care, and that the need for transportation to and from providers presented a barrier to children receiving Medicaid dental services.[1] Other research reiterates the effect that a lack of transportation can have on access. For example, one study cited an estimate that approximately 3.6 million Americans miss or delay care because they lack appropriate transportation to reach their medical appointments.[2] Another study noted that for poorer populations, which tend to encounter more barriers to accessing health care generally, transportation can be a significant issue to accessing care.[3] Given that transportation limitations can disproportionately affect low-income individuals' access to medical services, Medicaid's NEMT benefit can serve as an important safety net for program enrollees.

Under the Patient Protection and Affordable Care Act (PPACA), states can opt to expand eligibility for Medicaid to most non-elderly, nonpregnant adults who are not eligible for Medicare, and whose incomes are at or below 133 percent of the federal poverty level (FPL).[4] The decision whether to expand Medicaid can be a complex consideration for states, involving competing interests, as well as decisions about the structure and content of states' programs—such as the scope of benefits offered to newly eligible Medicaid enrollees. Although states are required to ensure necessary transportation to and from providers for newly eligible enrollees covered through their state plans, some states have received approval to expand Medicaid coverage through demonstration projects under section 1115 of the Social Security Act.[5] Under this authority, states may obtain a waiver to exclude the NEMT benefit for newly eligible enrollees.[6] As of September 2015, 30 states had expanded Medicaid eligibility, some through demonstrations.[7]

Given that states are making decisions about whether to expand Medicaid and how to structure their programs, you asked us to explore state efforts to exclude the NEMT benefit for newly eligible Medicaid enrollees. This report examines

1. the extent to which states have undertaken efforts to exclude the NEMT benefit for newly eligible enrollees; and
2. what is known about the potential implications of excluding the NEMT benefit on newly eligible enrollees' access to Medicaid services.

To examine the extent to which states have undertaken efforts to exclude the NEMT benefit for newly eligible enrollees, we interviewed officials from the Centers for Medicare & Medicaid Services (CMS) and contacted the 30 states that expanded Medicaid as of September 30, 2015. In the states that reported undertaking efforts to exclude the NEMT benefit, we interviewed Medicaid officials and reviewed relevant documents, including special terms and conditions associated with their demonstrations and related approval letters, if available.

To examine what is known about the potential implications of excluding the NEMT benefit on newly eligible enrollees' access to Medicaid services, we reviewed states' waiver evaluation designs, methodologies, and any related reports. Additionally, we evaluated the methodology that one state used in its evaluation of the effect of excluding NEMT for newly eligible Medicaid enrollees. We also interviewed CMS officials regarding their oversight of these states' efforts, including their role in assessing and approving them. In addition, based on referrals from subject-matter experts and knowledge of the organizations' roles related to Medicaid's NEMT benefit, we identified 10 national and local research and advocacy groups to interview, which included groups offering enrollee, underserved population, and provider perspectives on changes to the NEMT benefit. We also reviewed GAO and other research on transportation services for disadvantaged populations, and the role of transportation in the Medicaid expansion population's efforts to obtain health care services.

We conducted this performance audit from June 2015 to January 2016 in accordance with generally accepted government auditing standards. Those standards require that we plan and perform the audit to obtain sufficient, appropriate evidence to provide a reasonable basis for our findings and conclusions based on our audit objectives. We believe that the evidence obtained provides a reasonable basis for our findings and conclusions based on our audit objectives.

BACKGROUND

Within the Department of Health and Human Services (HHS), CMS is responsible for overseeing Medicaid at the federal level, while states are responsible for the day-to-day operations of their Medicaid programs. Under section 1115 of the Social Security Act, the Secretary of HHS may waive certain Medicaid requirements to allow states to implement demonstrations through which states can test and evaluate new approaches for delivering Medicaid services that, in the Secretary's judgment, are likely to assist in promoting Medicaid objectives.[8] Prior to the enactment of PPACA, states that wanted to expand Medicaid coverage to childless adults could do so only under a demonstration. While states may now expand their programs to cover these individuals through a state plan amendment, some states have expanded coverage under demonstrations in order to tailor coverage for this group in a manner that differs from what federal law requires. For example, states are not permitted to exclude coverage of mandatory benefits, such as NEMT, under their state plans, but they may do so by obtaining a waiver of the requirement under a demonstration.[9]

Recently, the Secretary of HHS approved various states' demonstrations to test alternative approaches, such as allowing states to use Medicaid funds to provide newly eligible enrollees with premium assistance to purchase private health plans in their respective state marketplace, or to exclude from coverage certain mandatory Medicaid benefits, such as NEMT, for newly eligible enrollees.[10] CMS has required those states that have obtained approval to exclude the NEMT benefit for one year under a demonstration to submit annual evaluations on the effect of this change on access to care, which will inform the agency's decision to approve any extension requests.

Evaluations by research organizations identified the lack of transportation as a barrier to care that can affect costs and health outcomes. For example, a survey of adults in the National Health Interview Survey found that limited transportation disproportionally affected Medicaid enrollees' access to primary care.[11] A study by the Transportation Research Board found that individuals who miss medical appointments due to transportation issues could potentially exacerbate diseases, thus leading to costly subsequent care, such as emergency room visits and hospitalizations.[12] We also previously reported that there are many federal programs, including Medicaid, that provide the NEMT benefit to the transportation-disadvantaged population.[13] However, in this work we found that coordination of NEMT programs at the federal level is limited, and there is fragmentation, overlap, and the potential for duplication across NEMT programs. As a result, individuals who rely on these programs may encounter fragmented services that are narrowly focused and difficult to navigate, possibly resulting in NEMT service gaps.[14]

State Efforts to Exclude Medicaid NEMT Benefits Are Not Widespread

Among the 30 states that expanded Medicaid as of September 30, 2015, 25 reported that they did not undertake efforts to exclude the NEMT benefit for newly eligible Medicaid enrollees and were not considering doing so.[15] Three states reported pursuing such efforts, and two states did not respond to our inquiry, although CMS indicated that neither of these states undertook efforts to exclude the NEMT benefit. (See fig. 1.)

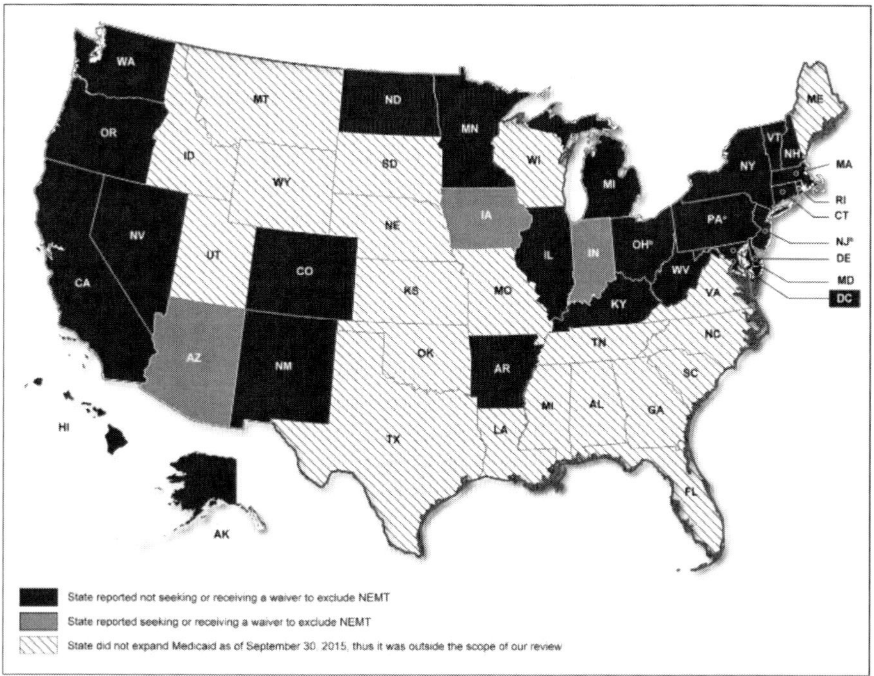

Source: State Medicaid officials. | GAO-16-221.

[a] As part of Pennsylvania's efforts to expand Medicaid under a demonstration, the state received approval to exclude the NEMT benefit for its newly eligible enrollees; however, the state ultimately did not implement this waiver. Thus, newly eligible enrollees remained eligible for the NEMT benefit.

[b] Although we did not receive responses from New Jersey and Ohio, the Centers for Medicare & Medicaid Services provided information about these states' efforts related to the NEMT benefit.

Figure 1. State-Reported Actions to Exclude Medicaid's Nonemergency Medical Transportation (NEMT) Benefit for Newly Eligible Enrollees, September 2015.

Three states (Indiana, Iowa, and Arizona) reported undertaking efforts to exclude the NEMT benefit under a demonstration as part of a broader health care initiative to expand Medicaid in their respective states. However, only

Indiana and Iowa had received approval from HHS for these waivers as of September 30, 2015, while Arizona was still seeking approval.

Indiana: Indiana's effort to exclude the NEMT benefit from coverage pre-dates PPACA and is not specific to newly eligible enrollees under the state's expansion. Beginning in February 2015, Indiana expanded Medicaid under a demonstration that provides two levels of coverage for newly eligible enrollees, depending on their income level and payment of premiums. As part of this demonstration, the state received approval to exclude the NEMT benefit for newly eligible enrollees. Indiana's efforts to implement its Medicaid expansion are based, in part, on another demonstration that the state has had in place since 2008.[16] Under this older demonstration, which provided authority for the state to offer Medicaid coverage to certain uninsured adults, NEMT was not a covered benefit for this population.

Iowa: Iowa expanded Medicaid in response to PPACA through two demonstrations beginning in January 2014. Under these demonstrations, the state offers two separate programs for newly eligible enrollees: one that offers Medicaid coverage administered by the state to enrollees with incomes up to 100 percent of the FPL, and a second that offers premium assistance to purchase private coverage through the state's health insurance marketplace for those enrollees with incomes from 100 to 133 percent of the FPL.[17] For both of these demonstrations, the state received approval to exclude the NEMT benefit. Similar to Indiana, Iowa's effort to exclude the NEMT benefit for a portion of its Medicaid population pre-dates PPACA. In July 2005, Iowa expanded Medicaid to certain populations under a demonstration with limited benefits that did not include NEMT.[18]

Arizona: When Arizona expanded Medicaid in January 2014, it had not sought to exclude the NEMT benefit for newly eligible enrollees. However, when the state submitted a request on September 30, 2015, to extend its longstanding demonstration, it sought approval to exclude the NEMT benefit.[19] Arizona's proposed extension would require newly eligible adults, including those with incomes from 100 to 133 percent of the FPL, to enroll in a new Medicaid program that includes enrollee contributions into an account that can be used for non-covered services and an employment incentive program.[20] The proposed extension, including the request to exclude the NEMT benefit, was under review, as of November 2015.

Officials from these three states cited several reasons for their efforts to exclude the NEMT benefit, including a desire to align Medicaid benefits with private insurance plans, which typically do not cover this benefit.

- Indiana officials indicated that when the state initially developed its demonstration in 2008, they designed benefits for a low-income population that tended to be employed. Thus, under that demonstration they offered benefits that resembled private insurance in an effort to familiarize enrollees with private coverage. This experience largely influenced the state's decision under its current demonstration to exclude the NEMT benefit for newly eligible enrollees.
- Iowa officials reported that when the state expanded Medicaid, they wanted Medicaid benefits to look like a private insurance plan—with the hope of limiting disruptions in service as fluctuations in income could result in changes to enrollees' coverage.
- While Arizona officials also cited the state's intent to align Medicaid benefits with private health insurance, they also noted that excluding the NEMT benefit would be one way to contain costs.

Of the remaining 25 Medicaid expansion states, 14 offered reasons for why they did not exclude the NEMT benefit for newly eligible enrollees.[21]

- Officials from 8 states reported they did not pursue such efforts because they considered the NEMT benefit critical to ensuring enrollees' access to care.
- Officials from an additional 4 states reported that they wanted to align benefits for the newly eligible enrollees with those offered to enrollees covered under the traditional Medicaid state plan.
- Officials from 2 other states reported that the newly eligible Medicaid enrollees did not significantly increase their program enrollment, and therefore, there was no need to alter this benefit.

TWO STATES ARE EVALUATING IMPLICATIONS OF EXCLUDING NEMT; RESEARCHERS AND ADVOCATES RAISED CONCERNS ABOUT ALTERING THE BENEFIT

The two states that excluded the NEMT benefit are in different stages of completing required evaluations of the effect of this exclusion on access to care. Research and advocacy groups indicated that excluding the NEMT benefit could affect enrollees' access to services and costs of coverage, and could set a precedent for the Medicaid program moving forward.

Evaluations of Efforts to Exclude the NEMT Benefit in Two States Assess Comparability of Access for Enrollees with and without Benefit

The two states that obtained approval to exclude the NEMT benefit for newly eligible Medicaid enrollees—Indiana and Iowa—are at different stages of evaluating the effect this will have on enrollees and have different time frames for reporting their results. Indiana officials indicated that the state is currently working with CMS on the design of its evaluation and must submit results to CMS by February 29, 2016.[22] According to a draft of the evaluation design, the state plans to survey enrollees and providers to compare the experiences of Medicaid enrollees with and without the NEMT benefit with respect to missed appointments, preventative care, and overall health outcomes; the state also seeks to determine whether enrollees residing in certain parts of the state are more affected by a lack of this benefit.[23]

Similarly, Iowa, which excluded the NEMT benefit for all newly eligible enrollees beginning in January 2014, was required to submit a series of independent analyses to CMS and recently received approval to continue its exclusion of this benefit until March 2016.[24] The state conducted an analysis to determine whether newly eligible enrollees' access to services was affected and reported its results in April 2015. Developed in close consultation with CMS, the analysis focused on the comparability of experiences of enrollees covered under the Medicaid state plan (who have the NEMT benefit) with newly eligible Medicaid expansion enrollees (who do not have the NEMT benefit).[25] With such a focus, the analysis sought to determine whether excluding the NEMT benefit presented more of a barrier to obtaining services than an enrollee would have otherwise experienced under the state's Medicaid state plan. Using enrollee surveys, the analysis found little difference in the barriers to care experienced by the two groups of enrollees as a result of transportation-related issues.[26] For example, the analysis noted that about 20 percent of enrollees in both groups reported usually or always needing help from others to get to a health care appointment.[27] Additionally, the analysis identified comparability between both groups of enrollees in terms of their reported unmet need for transportation to medical appointments (about 12 percent of both groups) and reported worry about the ability to pay for the associated costs (13 percent of both groups).

However, looking within the group of newly eligible enrollees without the NEMT benefit, the Iowa evaluation found that those with lower incomes—under 100 percent of the FPL—tended to need more transportation assistance and have more unmet needs than those with higher incomes. For example,

- 25 percent of newly eligible enrollees with incomes under 100 percent of the FPL reported needing help with transportation, compared with 11 percent of higher income newly eligible enrollees;
- 15 percent of newly eligible enrollees with incomes under 100 percent of the FPL reported an unmet need for transportation, compared with 5 percent of higher income newly eligible enrollees; and
- 14 percent of newly eligible enrollees with incomes under 100 percent of the FPL reported that they worried a lot about paying for transportation, compared with 6 percent of higher income newly eligible enrollees that reported that they worried a lot about paying for transportation.

HHS recently approved Iowa's amendment to continue its waiver of the NEMT benefit, although it noted concern about the lower income enrollees' experience. In approving the state's request, HHS cited the need for Iowa to continue evaluating the effects of the waiver in light of survey results on the type of transportation that newly eligible enrollees reported using to get to health care appointments. These results showed that newly eligible enrollees tended to rely on others, such as family and friends, to reach health care appointments more so than Medicaid state plan enrollees.[28]

Researchers who conducted the evaluation of Iowa's program indicated that they plan to conduct additional analyses, which include some—but not all—of the suggestions we have offered.[29] For example, our review of Iowa's evaluation methodology suggests that linking survey responses from both groups of enrollees directly to their claims could improve the state's understanding of enrollees' patterns of utilization and the implications of transportation difficulties. The researchers indicated that they will link claims data with survey responses in the next evaluation and use regression modeling to determine which group of enrollees was more likely to have an unmet need due to transportation issues. Additionally, we noted that the small sample size could limit their ability to detect differences between the enrollees. The researchers indicated that their next evaluation will survey a larger sample of

Medicaid enrollees covered under the state plan who have the NEMT benefit and newly eligible enrollees who do not in an effort to increase their ability to detect these differences. We agree that increasing the sample size could strengthen confidence in the results. We also noted that the researchers did not consider whether survey respondents lived in a rural or urban area, which can be important because research shows that the need to travel longer distances and the lack of public transportation in rural areas can pose challenges for individuals seeking services. The researchers indicated that they did not stratify the groups by rural or urban areas because of a concern about inadequate sample sizes in certain counties and because the need for transportation in Iowa is not unique to the pursuit of health care services, but also poses a challenge in other aspects of residents' lives.[30] While stratifying survey results by rural and urban areas could be relevant in evaluating enrollees' access to care or unmet need, the researchers do not plan to include a rural and urban stratification in the next evaluation.[31] CMS officials recognized the value of a rural and urban distinction, but indicated that there is a need to balance further analysis with the ability to generate results expeditiously and facilitate decision making on the waiver.

Research and Advocacy Groups Raised Concerns Regarding the Implications of Altering the Transportation Benefit for Newly Eligible Enrollees

Officials from the 10 research and advocacy groups we interviewed—which represent Medicaid enrollees, underserved populations, and health care providers—noted potential concerns of excluding the NEMT benefit as it relates to enrollee access to services and costs of coverage.

Access to Services: Officials from 9 of the 10 groups we interviewed indicated that excluding the NEMT benefit would impede newly eligible enrollees' ability to access health care services, particularly individuals living in rural or underserved areas, as well as those with chronic health conditions.[32] For example, officials from one national group that represents underserved populations indicated that the enrollees affected by the lack of the NEMT benefit will be those living in rural areas that must travel long distances for medical services. Another group that represents providers in Iowa also cited the difficulty faced by enrollees that live in rural areas by noting that some of the patients they served have had to cancel their medical appointments because the patients do not have a car, money to pay for gas, or access to public transportation. With respect to enrollees with chronic health conditions, one group that represents transportation providers (and others who support mobility efforts) noted that transportation can be a major barrier for individuals who are chronically ill and need recurring access to life-saving health services. Similarly, another group that represents community health centers specified that those with mental health conditions are particularly vulnerable due to a lack of transportation.[33]

Costs of Coverage: Officials from 5 of the 10 groups we interviewed also noted that efforts to exclude the NEMT benefit can have implications on the costs of care because patients without access to transportation may forgo preventive care or health services and end up needing more expensive care, such as ambulance services or emergency room visits. For example, a national group that represents providers of services for low-income populations noted that for people who are receiving regular substance abuse treatments, missing appointments can make them vulnerable to relapsing, which ultimately drives up the cost of their care. Another national group that represents underserved populations indicated that they have seen low-income individuals who do not have a car and cannot afford public transportation use higher-cost care from emergency rooms for their medical problems because they cannot otherwise access care. One other group that represents providers noted that by driving up the cost of care, a lack of transportation will ultimately trickle down to lower reimbursement rates for providers.

Despite these potential implications, officials from 9 of the 10 groups we interviewed acknowledged various advantages of a state expanding Medicaid even with a more limited benefit. For example, officials from 4 groups remarked that some coverage is better than no coverage in light of the significant health care needs among low-income populations. These groups recognized the political challenges that have driven state decisions whether to expand Medicaid and the concessions that are needed for an expansion to occur. For example, officials from a group that represents providers in Iowa indicated that although introducing variations in Medicaid programs adds complexity for providers, patients, and the state, flexibility is important in helping a state find a coverage solution that works in its political climate. Similarly, an advocacy group from one state acknowledged that an expansion with full traditional Medicaid benefits was never going to be achieved in that state, given the political environment. As such, groups within that state's provider community broadly supported the state's effort to expand Medicaid—even without the NEMT benefit—because so much of the population was uninsured and needed this coverage.

However, while acknowledging their preference for states to expand Medicaid, three groups we spoke with maintained their concerns about the effects of such efforts on enrollees' access to care. Officials from two of these groups said that improvements in the number of people covered should not be achieved by eroding essential services, while an official from the other group questioned the value of having health coverage if an enrollee is unable to get to the location where services are provided. Further, officials from six of the groups we interviewed were concerned that HHS's approvals of state efforts to exclude the NEMT benefit potentially provide other states with an incentive to pursue similar efforts.

These six groups raised concerns that every time HHS approves such an effort, a new baseline is created for what states may request in an effort to exclude core Medicaid services.[34]

AGENCY COMMENTS

We provided a draft of this report to HHS for comment. The department provided technical comments, which we incorporated as appropriate.

Carolyn L. Yocom
Director, Health Care

Mark L. Goldstein
Director, Physical Infrastructure

End Notes

[1] See GAO, Medicaid: States Made Multiple Program Changes, and Beneficiaries Generally Reported Access Comparable to Private Insurance, GAO-13-55 (Washington, D.C.: Nov. 15, 2012); and Medicaid: State and Federal Actions Have Been Taken to Improve Children's Access to Dental Services, but Gaps Remain, GAO-09-723 (Washington, D.C.: Sept. 30, 2009).

[2] See National Conference of State Legislatures, Non-Emergency Medical Transportation: A Vital Lifeline for a Health Community, January 2015.

[3] See J Community Health, Traveling Toward Disease: Transportation Barriers to Health Care Access, vol. 38, Issue 5 (October 2013), 976 – 993.

[4] PPACA also imposes a 5 percent income disregard when calculating modified adjusted gross income, which, in effect, raises this income limit to 138 percent of the FPL.

[5] A Medicaid state plan is an agreement between a state and the federal government describing how that state administers its Medicaid program. When a state wishes to make a change to its program policies or operational approach, it may submit a state plan amendment that is reviewed for approval by CMS.

[6] States that wish to alter their Medicaid programs in ways that depart from federal requirements may seek approval to implement Medicaid demonstration projects under section 1115 of the Social Security Act. This provision authorizes the Secretary of Health and Human Services (HHS) to waive certain federal Medicaid requirements and allow costs that would not otherwise be eligible for federal matching funds for experimental, pilot, or demonstration projects that, in the Secretary's judgment, are likely to assist in promoting Medicaid objectives. See 42 U.S.C. § 1315(a). For example, states may seek a waiver of Medicaid's NEMT regulation, which requires state plans to ensure necessary transportation for beneficiaries to and from providers. See 42 C.F.R. § 431.53. In this report, we use the term "demonstration" to refer to state demonstration projects authorized by CMS under section 1115, whereas we use the term "waiver" when referring to waivers of the NEMT requirement under such a demonstration.

[7] For purposes of this report, "state" includes the District of Columbia. Montana has also opted to expand Medicaid, but its expansion does not go into effect until January 1, 2016.

[8] See 42 U.S.C. § 1315(a). Generally, demonstrations are approved for an initial 5-year period and can be extended for additional years.

[9] While state plans may not exclude coverage of NEMT services, states may place appropriate limits on a service based on such criteria as medical necessity or on utilization control procedures. See 42 C.F.R. § 440.230(d). For example, CMS approved a state plan amendment in Arkansas that requires most newly eligible Medicaid enrollees to obtain prior authorization after eight NEMT trips. According to Arkansas officials, after the eighth trip, such enrollees must call into the designated NEMT contractor and answer a series of questions to demonstrate their need for transportation. This prior authorization requirement does not apply to newly eligible Medicaid enrollees that are deemed medically frail, which account for about 10 percent of the state's newly eligible enrollees, according to Arkansas officials. States have some flexibility to define who is medically frail; however, they must, at a minimum, include individuals who have (1) disabling mental disorders; (2) chronic substance use disorders; (3) serious and complex medical conditions; (4) a disability determination based on Social Security criteria or more restrictive state criteria, if applicable; or individuals (5) who are described in 42 C.F.R. § 438.50(d)(3), such as those who are dually eligible. 42 C.F.R. 440.315(f).

[10] Marketplaces are a single point-of-access for individuals to enroll in private health insurance plans and apply for income-based financial assistance.

[11] Cheung, P., J. Wiler, R. Lowe, A. Ginde, "National Study of Barriers to Timely Primary Care and Emergency Department Utilization Among Medicaid Beneficiaries," Annals of Emergency Medicine (July 2012).

[12] Transit Cooperative Research Program, Cost Benefit Analysis of Providing Non-Emergency Medical Transportation, October 2005, accessed on September 15, 2015, http://online pubs.trb.org/onlinepubs/tcrp /tcrp_webdoc_29.pdf.

[13] The transportation-disadvantaged population generally includes those individuals who cannot provide their own transportation due to age, disability, or income constraints.

[14] For example, see GAO, Transportation Disadvantaged Populations: Nonemergency Medical Transportation Not Well Coordinated, and Additional Federal Leadership Needed, GAO-15-110 (Washington, D.C.: Dec. 10, 2014); and Transportation Disadvantaged Populations:

Federal Coordination Efforts Could be Further Strengthened, GAO-12-647 (Washington, D.C.: June 20, 2012).

[15] As part of Pennsylvania's efforts to expand Medicaid under a demonstration, the state received approval to exclude the NEMT benefit for its newly eligible enrollees; however, the state ultimately did not implement this waiver. Thus, newly eligible enrollees remained eligible for the NEMT benefit.

[16] Indiana's Medicaid expansion is called the Healthy Indiana Plan (HIP) 2.0—which is based, in part, on a previous section 1115 demonstration called HIP 1.0. While HIP 1.0 covered certain health services, it did not offer the NEMT benefit to enrollees.

[17] Iowa's Medicaid expansion is called the Iowa Health and Wellness Plan. Within this program, enrollees with incomes under 100 percent of the FPL are enrolled in the Wellness Plan, and enrollees with incomes from 101 to 138 percent of the FPL are enrolled in the Marketplace Choice Plan. Because there is only one health plan participating in the program, Marketplace Choice enrollees, as of December 2014, are no longer required to enroll in premium assistance as a condition of eligibility, but may choose to participate in the Wellness Plan.

[18] Iowa's 2005 demonstration—called IowaCare—provided Medicaid coverage for individuals aged 19 through 64 with incomes up to 200 percent of the FPL and pregnant women with incomes up to 300 percent of the FPL who have incurred medical expenses that reduced their income to 200 percent of the FPL. This demonstration also required enrollees to obtain services from certain provider networks.

[19] Since 1982, Arizona has offered Medicaid coverage through a demonstration that established the Arizona Health Care Cost Containment System. This demonstration allowed Arizona to mandate managed care, provide long term care services in home and community-based settings, and implement administrative simplifications, among other things. It is scheduled to expire on September 30, 2016.

[20] Arizona's demonstration application specifically excludes from the NEMT benefit waiver individuals with a serious mental illness, American Indians and Alaska Natives, individuals who are medically frail (to be defined through discussion with CMS), and individuals who serve as caregivers to an individual who is elderly or disabled. Similarly, Indiana's and Iowa's approved waivers of the NEMT benefit exempt individuals that the states define as medically frail.

[21] While we did not specifically ask officials in these 25 states for the reasons that they did not seek to exclude the NEMT benefit for newly eligible Medicaid enrollees, 14 states offered reasons for their decisions to maintain the benefit.

[22] In working with the state, CMS recently approved a temporary extension of the NEMT waiver through November 30, 2016.

[23] Indiana officials indicated that because the state had excluded the NEMT benefit for a segment of its Medicaid population since 2008 under its initial demonstration, it had already studied the effect that this waiver had on enrollees' access to services. In a 2012 survey conducted by researchers retained by the state, 800 enrollees were asked why they had not visited a doctor for a routine check-up in the last 12 months and 2.33 percent of respondents indicated that it takes too long to get there or they had a transportation problem in 2012.

[24] The state contracted with the University of Iowa, Public Policy Center to conduct this analysis. Researchers from the Public Policy Center indicated that they have worked with Iowa's Department of Human Services on a number of evaluations for 25 years—and thus have developed expertise with the state's Medicaid administrative claims and enrollment data.

[25] Researchers from the Public Policy Center told us that they worked closely with CMS for 6 months to develop the evaluation methodology, and although Iowa Medicaid officials were included in the meetings with CMS, they generally did not participate in the methodological discussions. Additionally, the researchers noted that under its contract with the state, the state is provided 30 days to review the Public Policy Center's report for accuracy, but does not have the ability to edit the content.
For the results of Iowa's evaluations, see The University of Iowa Public Policy Center, Evaluation of the Iowa Health and Wellness Plan, Member Experiences in the First Year (April 2015); The University of Iowa Public Policy Center, Non-emergency Transportation Services for IHAWP Members: The Early Experiences of Iowa Health and Wellness Plan Members, A Policy Brief (March 2015); and The University of Iowa Public Policy Center, First Look at Iowa's Medicaid Expansion: How Well Did Members Transition to the Iowa Health and Wellness Plan from IowaCare (October 2014).

[26] The Iowa analysis also included a geographical assessment of distance to primary care providers based on a geocoding/mapping technique. To compare Medicaid state plan enrollees and newly eligible enrollees with incomes under 100 percent of the FPL, enrollees in both groups with at least one claim for preventive care were mapped to the provider who provided this care, and those without a claim for services were mapped to the closest primary care provider. The results from this analysis indicate no practical difference in the distance to a primary care provider in miles or minutes between newly eligible enrollees and enrollees under the state plan.

[27] Specifically, survey results indicated that about 20 percent of enrollees with the NEMT benefit and 22 percent of newly eligible enrollees without the NEMT benefit reported usually or always needing help from other sources to get to health care appointments.

[28] See HHS approval letter dated July 31, 2015.

[29] The researchers emphasized that the evaluation was not specific to the NEMT benefit, but was an evaluation of the impact of the state's entire 1115 demonstration. The researchers acknowledged that if their focus was on the NEMT benefit, they may have structured the survey questions and analyses differently. They further noted that in their continued evaluation, keeping the questions similar to those asked previously will allow them to compare the results over time.

[30] Additionally, the researchers noted that they are not considering stratifying results by rural and urban location, in part, because the evaluation is focused on whether there are any differences in experiences between the comparison groups and not on who is or is not receiving the NEMT benefit.

[31] The researchers indicated that they plan to survey about 30,000 enrollees, which will consist of those in the Medicaid state plan who have the NEMT benefit and the newly eligible who do not, and report the results to CMS in the spring of 2016. This is a larger sample than the previous survey, which consisted of 4,050 Medicaid state plan enrollees with the NEMT benefit and 6,750 enrollees without it. For the prior survey, 19 percent of the enrollees with the NEMT benefit responded to the survey, while 30 percent of enrollees without the NEMT benefit responded.

[32] While certain newly eligible enrollees with chronic conditions in Indiana and Iowa may qualify for the NEMT benefit by being determined medically frail, officials from some of the groups we spoke with cited limitations in terms of who can qualify as medically frail, as well as long wait times for such determinations.

[33] We previously cited Substance Abuse and Mental Health Administration estimates that approximately 3 million (17 percent) of the 17.8 million low-income, uninsured adults

nationwide had a behavioral health condition prior to the Medicaid expansion in 2014. See GAO, Behavioral Health: Options for Low-income Adults to Receive Treatment in Selected States, GAO-15-449 (Washington, D.C.: June 19, 2015).

[34] In particular, officials from two of the six groups pointed to Arizona's recent request to exclude the NEMT benefit from coverage for newly eligible enrollees. Arizona had not sought to do so when it initially expanded Medicaid under its demonstration, but then pursued this option after other states were approved to do so.

In: Nonemergency Medical Transportation ISBN: 978-1-53610-118-8
Editor: Trevor Davis

Chapter 3

LET MEDICAID GIVE YOU A RIDE*

Centers for Medicare & Medicaid Services

Medicaid covers the cost of emergency medical transportation for eligible individuals. An emergency is when your medical needs are immediate. Examples include having a heart attack or being seriously injured in a car accident. In cases like these, you may be taken to the emergency room by ground (ambulance) or air (medical flight). You do not need pre-approval for emergency transportation. If you need a ride to a medical appointment, Medicaid does not consider this an emergency, but you may still be able to get a ride.

Medicaid covers rides for eligible individuals to and from the doctor's office, the hospital, or another medical office for Medicaid-approved care. This coverage is called "non-emergency medical transportation," because it does not involve a medical emergency. Medicaid may give you a ride if you do not have a car that works or do not have a driver's license. You may also be able to get a ride if you have a physical or mental disability or are unable to travel or wait for a ride alone. Coverage for these rides may be different depending on your individual situation and needs. You may need to get your State Medicaid agency's approval to qualify for a ride.

* This is an edited, reformatted and augmented version of a fact sheet issued April 2016.

Who Can Get a Ride?

Federal regulations say that Medicaid beneficiaries can get rides to and from providers when necessary [1]. States have different rules about when rides are necessary, so make sure you check with your State. Generally, when you enroll in Medicaid, you will receive instructions about when a ride is necessary and how and when you can schedule a ride. You may have to call a Medicaid caseworker, a ride service, or another agency. That contact should:

- Help you decide if you have an immediate need for care;
- Make sure you are eligible for Medicaid;
- Verify that you have an appointment with a Medicaid provider;
- Make sure that you have no other reasonable way to make it to your appointment; and
- Decide what type of ride Medicaid can give you for your situation.

Based on this information, your contact will either set up the ride you need or will tell you how to set up the ride yourself. A person or ride service approved by the State Medicaid program will take you to and from your appointment [2].

Generally, if you are enrolled in a Medicaid managed care plan, the customer service staff can give you facts about ride benefits.

How Do I Get a Ride?

Depending on your needs and your State's rules, rides might be by taxi, car, van, public bus, or a subway. You might share your ride with others. You have to call to set up your ride in advance, and you should call if you need to cancel. Remember, the driver can give you or an eligible family member a ride only to a medical office and back home. If the driver gives you a ride anywhere else, you and the driver could be charged with stealing from Medicaid.

Make sure to follow the rules so Medicaid will approve and pay for your ride. Drivers may be authorized only for specific times to pick up the rider. It is important to:

- Be ready on time for the pickup; and

- Call the ride service to cancel a scheduled ride if you do not need the ride anymore.

In some places, Medicaid might not pay ride services for the time a driver waits for you to arrive or if you do not show up for planned pickups. In other States, there may be limits on how long the driver can wait for you if you are not on time. If you make a habit of not showing up for scheduled rides, you may have to make extra calls to the ride service to verify that you intend to keep your appointment. Medicaid may also place additional restrictions on your ability to get a ride, like requiring you to use only one service to get your rides.

What If My Ride Does Not Show Up?

What should you do if your ride does not show up? Call the number you used to set up your ride. Stay calm and explain the problem. The ride service should help you. Then call your medical provider, and explain it to them.

What If My Appointment Is Changed?

If your appointment is changed, call your ride service as soon as you can. Explain why you are changing your ride time and set up a new pickup time.

What Happens If the Rules Are Not Followed?

If providers and beneficiaries do not follow the rules for Medicaid, the added cost to the Medicaid program can be significant. Fraud and abuse can affect the amount of money available for Medicaid benefits. Help prevent fraud by reporting an incident when:

- Your driver takes someone to a nonmedical location other than their home;
- Your driver takes a route that adds extra time or mileage;
- You get a ride in an ambulance when a wheelchair or regular van would have worked; or

- You see someone sharing his or her Medicaid card or number with others to get medical services.

These are just some examples of fraud. If you know of someone who is breaking the rules, including a driver, report it.

Fraud and Abuse: How Do I Report Them?

You can report fraud anonymously, but it is helpful to give your phone number or email address so an investigator can contact you for more information. If you do give your contact information, the investigators will protect your identity to the maximum extent provided by the law.

Report fraud to your State Medicaid Fraud Control Unit or State Medicaid agency. Their contact information is available at https://www.cms.gov/medicare-medicaid-coordination/fraud-prevention/fraudabuseforconsumers/report_fraud_and_suspected_fraud.html on the Centers for Medicare & Medicaid Services (CMS) website, or contact the U.S. Department of Health and Human Services, Office of Inspector General.

Office of Inspector General
U.S. Department of Health and Human Services
ATTN: Hotline
P.O. Box 23489
Washington, DC 20026
Phone: 1-800-HHS-TIPS (1-800-447-8477)
TTY: 1-800-377-4950
Fax: 1-800-223-8164
Email: HHSTips@oig.hhs.gov
Website: https://forms.oig.hhs.gov/hotlineoperations/

To see the electronic version of this fact sheet and the other products included in the "Non-Emergency Medical Transportation" Toolkit, visit the Medicaid Program Integrity Education page at https://www.cms.gov/Medicare-Medicaid-Coordination/Fraud-Prevention/Medicaid-Integrity-Education/edmic-landing.html on the CMS website.

REFERENCES

[1] Assurance of Transportation, 42 C.F.R. § 431.53. Retrieved March 15, 2016, from http://www.ecfr.gov/cgi-bin/text-idx?c=ecfr&SID=cdb6a478293ced6a5371b84531517f63&rgn=div8&view=text&node=42:4.0.1.1.2.2.10.5&idno=42.

[2] Health Care Financing Administration. National Association of Medicaid Directors' Non-Emergency Transportation Technical Advisory Group. (1998, August). Designing and Operating Cost Effective Medicaid Non-Emergency Transportation Programs: A Guidebook for State Medicaid Agencies. Retrieved March 15, 2016, from http://ntl.bts.gov/lib/12000/12200/12290/medicaid.pdf.

In: Nonemergency Medical Transportation ISBN: 978-1-53610-118-8
Editor: Trevor Davis

Chapter 4

MEDICAID NON-EMERGENCY MEDICAL TRANSPORTATION BOOKLET FOR PROVIDERS*

Centers for Medicare & Medicaid Services

CONTENT SUMMARY

Medicaid non-emergency medical transportation (NEMT) is an important benefit for beneficiaries who need to get to and from medical services but have no means of transportation. The Code of Federal Regulations requires States to ensure that eligible, qualified Medicaid beneficiaries have NEMT to take them to and from providers. However, every State's Medicaid program is different. In addition, each State has the option of developing and implementing Medicaid waiver programs, which can provide coverage for additional transportation needs. Waiver program rules can also vary from State to State and even within the same State's programs. Providers are responsible for knowing and abiding by the specific rules for each State where they furnish services, and for each of the programs for which they furnish services. The booklet cites State-specific examples to illustrate the rule discussed.

This booklet summarizes the general scope of Medicaid-covered emergency transportation and NEMT benefits and reviews principles applicable to such coverage. It also explains three modes for States to

---

* This is an edited, reformatted and augmented version of a document issued April 2016.

provide or arrange for covered NEMT, common Medicaid transportation fraud and abuse issues, and provider tips to help prevent fraud and abuse. In addition, the booklet encourages providers to regularly check that their employees and contractors are not excluded from Federal health care programs.

Qualifying for Medicaid Non-Emergency Medical Transportation

The Code of Federal Regulations (CFR) requires States to "specify that the Medicaid agency will ensure necessary transportation for beneficiaries to and from providers;" and "describe the methods that the agency will use to meet this requirement"[1]. For situations that do not involve an immediate threat to the life or health of an individual, this requirement is usually called "non-emergency medical transportation," or NEMT.

For this booklet, an eligible beneficiary is defined as "an individual who has been determined eligible and is currently receiving Medicaid"[2]. For most individuals, these eligibility determinations are based on means-testing, by comparing an individual's income and, for some individuals, assets against an income or resource standard. Individuals with income or resources below the standard are determined eligible. Means-testing is an objective way to determine whether someone meets the criteria for Medicaid benefits.

When beneficiaries are eligible for Medicaid benefits, they may or may not qualify for NEMT services. To qualify, States may require that there be an unmet transportation need [3, 4]. Depending on State law, a qualifying unmet need can include:

- Not having a valid driver's license;
- Not having a working vehicle available in the household;
- Being unable to travel or wait for services alone; or
- Having a physical, cognitive, mental, or developmental limitation [5].

EMERGENCY AND NON-EMERGENCY MEDICAL TRANSPORTATION DEFINED

An emergency is any event that puts the health and life of a Medicaid beneficiary at serious risk without immediate treatment. Real emergencies occur when the medical needs of a beneficiary are immediate and due to severe symptoms. A life-threatening event such as uncontrolled bleeding, heart attack, an automobile accident, or other serious trauma may cause the symptoms.[6] Medicaid reimburses emergency transportation providers when they furnish services to eligible beneficiaries according to the rules.

The Medicaid NEMT benefit is authorized under the Social Security Act section 1902(a)(70) and 42 CFR section 440.170. Medicaid NEMT is transportation for eligible Medicaid beneficiaries to and from appointments and services for those who have a legitimate need for the services [7, 8]. At a minimum, a State Medicaid agency (SMA) or its designated managed care entity must:

- Ensure necessary transportation to and from providers;
- Use the most appropriate form of transportation; [9] and
- Include coverage for transportation and related travel expenses necessary to secure medical examinations and treatment [10].

As an NEMT provider, be sure to know the specific Medicaid rules for NEMT and any general State licensing or certification requirements for vehicles and drivers in the States where you furnish services, as they can be different from State to State. Most States publish a provider transportation manual. If you have questions or concerns, call the SMA for assistance.

Links to each SMA website, where specific questions and concerns can be answered, may be found at https://medicaid. gov/Medicaid-CHIP-Program-Information/By-State/By-State.html on the Medicaid website. States are invested in making sure that services are appropriate and furnished in accordance with Medicaid rules, that beneficiary needs are met, and that providers are paid correctly.

Contract Agreement

States can manage the authorization of NEMT coverage or contract with another entity to manage NEMT coverage, such as a transportation broker or a managed care organization.[11] Regardless of who manages NEMT coverage, Medicaid rules require the transportation provider to have a contract with the appropriate entity before any services are furnished [12]. If the provider is not under contract, Medicaid payment will not be available even if all of the other requirements for NEMT have been met.

Prior Authorization

Once a provider has a contract agreement, many States require coverage of transportation services to be preauthorized before the beneficiaries receive transportation. States preauthorize transportation in a variety of ways. For example, one State may expect a physician to authorize the need for beneficiary transportation, another State may only want to know that the beneficiary's location drop-off was to a medical appointment, while a third State may expect the medical facility to phone in the medical transportation request before providing services [13]. Each State establishes its own preauthorization rules.

Loaded Mileage

State Medicaid payment rules may take into account loaded mileage, location, and wait times. States and contracted transportation entities may only pay fee-for-service transportation providers for loaded mileage (a managed care entity may be paid a per member per month fee [pmpm]). A typical SMA definition of loaded mileage is the time a beneficiary is actually in the vehicle [14]. If a driver arrives at a preauthorized destination for pickup and transport and the beneficiary does not show up for the appointment, then that person is a no-show, and the provider generally cannot bill for the trip. Claiming loaded mileage when the beneficiary was a no-show is a common form of fraud in NEMT, and is an illegal practice [15]. It is called "billing for services not rendered" and may be prosecuted under the False Claims Act.

Location

State Medicaid rules may require beneficiaries to be picked up at home and taken to their medical services, and then be dropped off at home after they receive services. If a trip is to a nonmedical destination like the grocery store, shopping mall, to meet a friend, or something similar, State Medicaid rules do not cover the trip. Do not bill the trip to the Medicaid agency [16].

Wait Times

Finally, providers need to know that in most States, they cannot receive additional payment based on wait times. The costs of wait times may have been taken into account in determining overhead costs in setting transportation payment rates. Check with the State or the managing entity for any mandatory wait times in your State [17].

TYPES OF TRANSPORTATION

The different types of vehicles that providers can use for beneficiary transport to and from covered medical services include wheelchair vans, taxis, stretcher cars, and buses. In addition, providers can use other transportation determined appropriate by the SMA. For example, other transportation options might include air transportation or an ambulette [18].

TRANSPORTATION SERVICE DELIVERY SYSTEMS

There are different types of systems States can use to ensure non-emergency transportation for eligible Medicaid beneficiaries. This booklet discusses three of those systems. The three systems are: a transportation broker, transportation as a managed care benefit, and non-preauthorized contractors or vendors.

Transportation Broker

A Medicaid transportation broker contracts with an SMA to manage preauthorized NEMT services in a designated area. The broker bids for the opportunity to manage these services. The potential brokers submit bids, and the SMA evaluates them and choses brokers based on their "experience, performance, references, resources, qualifications, and costs" [19]. States hold nongovernmental brokers accountable to their contracts and the State Medicaid rules through regular audits and monitoring.

Once a broker has obtained an NEMT contract, they must "ensure that transport personnel are licensed, qualified, competent, and courteous" [20]. This is true for any Medicaid provider that hires drivers, not just brokers.

Not all States use brokers to ensure NEMT services. Some States retain the responsibility for qualifying and authorizing beneficiaries for transportation and then contract with one or more entities to furnish the transportation services.

Transportation as a Managed Care Benefit

States may contract with a managed care plan (MCP) that is then responsible for beneficiary transportation. The MCP must meet requirements for network sufficiency, solvency, and all other managed care requirements.

Non-Preauthorized Contractor or Vendor

States can also contract with independent transportation providers. These transportation providers must be qualified to provide the transportation under applicable State law. These transportation providers may include public transit options (buses, subway), professional drivers (taxis, limousines, vans), or volunteer drivers (family, friends, State-approved volunteers).

DRIVER CRITERIA

Depending on the State, there may be special criteria drivers must meet before they transport Medicaid beneficiaries. First, they must have the appropriate, current licenses for the types of vehicles they drive when transporting others. For example, States may require a chauffeur's license (or equivalent) for taxis and vans.

Second, a State may have qualifications for drivers that exceed the minimum to ensure that Medicaid beneficiaries receive a high quality of transportation. Standards might include limiting the number of points drivers can have against their license [21], certifying the health of a driver [22], carrying vehicle liability insurance [23], or having a criminal background check [24]. A recent OIG report found that some NEMT providers in one State had not completed the required online criminal background check [25].

Drivers should be required to treat beneficiaries with courtesy and respect. The State, the broker, or the transportation company should monitor any complaints made by beneficiaries related to access and quality—including any complaints received about the driver's behavior—and hold drivers accountable. In several States, two of the more frequent complaints about transportation providers concern the timeliness of the driver and the driver not showing up. Other top complaints include problems with the driver's behavior and "other stakeholders" [26, 27, 28].

Vehicle Criteria

It is important for transportation providers to remember that there may also be specific vehicle documentation and maintenance requirements [29, 30]. States may, for example, require providers to have documented proof the vehicle belongs to the correct entity and the identification number matches the ownership papers; the vehicle is legally licensed; the vehicle license plate is on the correct vehicle; and the vehicle is in good condition, safe for transport, and receives regular maintenance [31]. In addition, the State may require proof the vehicle has the current State-required liability insurance.

Fraud and Abuse Defined

Most transportation providers are honest and want to do the right thing. For example, a recent OIG report on California NEMT services outside of Los Angeles County found that 89 percent of sampled claims were compliant [32]. On the other hand, there are providers billing fraudulent, wasteful, or abusive claims. A provider must return any payment it receives for an improper claim to the SMA. Properly billing claims is the responsibility of everyone involved with Medicaid services. Brokers, providers, and drivers are all accountable for following Medicaid rules. Failure to comply with Medicaid transportation rules can result in penalties, fines, and prosecution, as previously discussed. Take the time to learn the definitions of fraud and abuse, understand common transportation schemes, and learn tips for preventing fraud and abuse. Check to ensure Federal health care programs do not exclude employees and contractors.

Medicaid rules define fraud as "an intentional deception or misrepresentation made by a person with the knowledge that the deception could result in some unauthorized benefit to himself or some other person" [33]. Fraudulent practices include billing for mileage when a beneficiary is not in the vehicle and billing for services that were never furnished.

Abuse is different from fraud. The Medicaid rules define abuse as practices "inconsistent with sound fiscal, business, or medical practices, and result in an unnecessary cost to the Medicaid program, or in reimbursement for services that are not medically necessary or that fail to meet professionally recognized standards for health care" [34].

FRAUD SCHEMES AND RESULTS

Any person or group of persons committing fraudulent acts can be held accountable. Fraudulent acts can include a variety of simple or elaborate schemes, as illustrated by the following examples.

Independent Contractor—Parent

Some States reimburse parents, considered independent contractors, for the cost of medically necessary trips. For example, a woman in Idaho was State-approved to regularly transport her child from their home in Idaho Falls, Idaho, to Salt Lake City for necessary medical treatment. However, in late 2007 through 2010, she began billing for trips that never occurred.

The State Attorney General's Medicaid Fraud Control Unit (MFCU) filed criminal charges against her. She was charged with three counts of Medicaid provider fraud and one count of grand theft. She pleaded guilty to two Medicaid fraud charges for falsifying her medical trip records and for receiving payment for the claims billed. On June 4, 2012, she was sentenced to jail. In addition to jail time and 5 years of probation, she was ordered to pay fines, restitution, and investigative costs of roughly $21,500 [35].

Beneficiary Fraud

A beneficiary who transported himself to dialysis treatments pleaded guilty to conspiring with an ambulance company owner to allow him to bill Medicaid for ambulance transportation for his dialysis appointments. The beneficiary even signed ambulance run sheets and transported other patients to dialysis in his own vehicle while the ambulance company owner billed for ambulance transportation for those people as well. The beneficiary also received kickbacks for referring other patients to the ambulance service [36].

Company Owner: Services Not Rendered

Providers should only bill for services rendered. If a beneficiary fails to show for a transportation appointment, a provider cannot bill Medicaid for the no-show. Nor should providers misuse beneficiary information to claim services they never provided. The owner of an Indiana NEMT company was found guilty of billing for services never provided, including billing for cancelled trips, upcoding some trips, and using patients' medical identifiers without their knowledge to bill for services they never received. The fraud scheme resulted in a loss of over $1 million to Indiana Medicaid [37].

Providers must use the most cost-effective mode of transportation when transporting Medicaid beneficiaries. They normally use ambulettes for transporting beneficiaries with a disability or for those who are convalescing and need additional care. Beneficiaries who use a wheelchair may be transported by ambulette. It is cost prohibitive to use ambulettes for those who do not need them. In May 2015, the owner of an ambulance company was sentenced to 6 months in jail and ordered to repay $200,000 to Medicaid. For 4 years, the owner had modified transportation request forms for a taxi to make it appear the patients needed the more expensive ambulette transportation.

Company—Qualified Drivers

Drivers must be qualified to transport Medicaid beneficiaries. Otherwise, the services are ineligible for reimbursement. On May 1, 2012, a Wisconsin specialized medical vehicle transportation company was convicted of falsifying drivers' records. The company documented that its drivers were trained and certified to furnish the services rendered to Medicaid beneficiaries. Former employees testified that the documentation was false.

The company was convicted of 18 counts of medical assistance fraud and ordered to pay a $10,000 fine and court costs [38].

Company Owner—Unauthorized Vehicles

Vehicles must be qualified when transporting Medicaid beneficiaries. A New York ambulette company owner was sentenced to 6 months in jail and 5 years' probation for modifying NEMT authorizations for taxi rides to ambulette services, which were 4 times more expensive. In addition to his sentencing, he also made full restitution of the $200,000 he stole from Medicaid [39, 40].

Taxi Driver

Beneficiaries who qualify for transportation services may only use the services for medically necessary appointments. Providers may not be reimbursed for services, even if they are furnished, if the services do not meet Medicaid rules (for example, dropping beneficiaries off at the grocery store or at a friend's home).

On December 18, 2012, a taxi driver in Alaska was convicted for violating Medicaid rules by taking beneficiaries to locations other than medical appointments, purchasing unused vouchers from investigators, and submitting vouchers for reimbursement that did not reflect the actual services he furnished.

The Anchorage driver was convicted of committing medical assistance fraud and ordered to pay a $500 fine and restitution. He was also sentenced to 3 years of probation and received a lifetime ban from billing for Medicaid-furnished services [41]. This action is called termination from a State Medicaid program. Providers who are excluded from one State's Medicaid program must also, by law, be excluded from all States' Medicaid programs as well as from Medicare programs nationwide.

FRAUD AND ABUSE PREVENTION TIPS

Preventing Medicaid transportation fraud is the responsibility of all providers. Providers should, within the scope of their authority and job duties, document the information the State wants, document furnished services completely and accurately, verify services were furnished according to the documentation, and bill correctly. For example, brokers, company owners, and drivers each have documentation responsibilities and should be sure their documentation is complete and accurate. Only brokers and owners have responsibility for verifying services were furnished according to what was documented.

Tip 1: Document Completely and Accurately, and Maintain Records

The Social Security Act requires all Medicaid providers to keep records and furnish them to the State upon request [42]. Each State determines what must be documented, and providers are responsible for keeping the information and producing it if the State asks for it. Transportation brokers and companies typically have their own documentation requirements in addition to what the State wants. To make sure they document records accordingly, providers will want to develop and implement specific transportation policies and procedures and see that their drivers are fully trained to meet the expectations.

Policies and procedures should emphasize the importance of drivers documenting records accurately and completely and include disciplinary action, up to and including termination, for falsifying transportation records. The main goals of documentation are to submit claims that represent the services furnished and to justify the claims billed. To meet these goals, records should be accurate and complete.

At a minimum, all States require providers to document the beneficiary's name and Medicaid identifier, the pickup and drop-off locations, the date and time the services were furnished, and the number of miles traveled with the beneficiary in the vehicle. Drivers should only document the number of loaded miles, as discussed previously.

Although there is no Federal rule requiring it, some States require transportation records to be in ink instead of pencil [43]. Some providers furnish drivers with printed computer sheets and allow them to document information directly on the sheets. If you do this, include this process in your policy, so if audited, the auditor understands why there is written information on the computer-generated documents [44].

Remember, if a service is not documented, there is no point in submitting a claim for reimbursement.

Tip 2: Verify Services

Some States and brokers require drivers to obtain the beneficiary's signature on the transport record at the end of the trip [45]. Even if the beneficiary's signature is required, it is the responsibility of management or a designee to verify documented services were furnished according to the record [46]. Do this by making random calls to beneficiaries listed on the record, and to personnel at the medical appointment location verifying beneficiary arrival and services.

Tip 3: Bill Accurately

Once services are verified, they can be billed. The claims submitted must reflect the actual services furnished. Providers normally bill State transportation services on the Centers for Medicare & Medicaid Services Form-1500 (CMS-1500). Instructions for the CMS-1500 include the following NOTICE: "Any person who knowingly files a statement of claim containing any misrepresentation of any false, incomplete or misleading information may be guilty of a criminal act punishable under law and may be subject to civil penalties" [47], so be sure to code claims correctly and represent the services furnished. Be sure to teach drivers not to embellish their records. This is for their own well-being.

CMS offers guidelines for claims submission:

- Use an original red-ink-on-white-paper CMS-1500 claim form;
- Use dark ink on the form;

- Use lift-off correction tape if making corrections to the form;
- Avoid handwritten, printed, or stamped information on the form;
- Make sure there are no staples, clips, or tape on the claim form;
- Remove any perforated edges on the claim form; and
- Include any required documentation with the claim form [48].

Check for Excluded Individuals and Parties

Providers should take one final action to protect themselves and their businesses from improper billings. Providers need to have a policy and procedure in place to check for excluded individuals and parties. As part of doing business, providers should make it part of policy and procedure to be diligent in screening all employees and contractors before hiring or contracting with them, and repeat the checks monthly to determine whether they are excluded from participation in Federal health care programs [49, 50]. The U.S. Department of Health and Human Services, Office of Inspector General (HHS-OIG) has the authority to exclude individuals and entities from participating in Federal programs for various reasons. Reasons include being convicted of certain crimes, losing one's license for lack of professional competence or financial integrity, or engaging in conduct prohibited by Medicaid rules [51]. When HHS-OIG excludes individuals or entities from participation, it places their names on the List of Excluded Individuals and Entities (LEIE) [52]. In the past, providers were also encouraged to check the Excluded Parties List System (EPLS). This has been replaced by the Exclusions Extract on the System for Award Management (SAM).

SAM combines the Federal procurement systems and the Catalog of Federal Domestic Assistance into one new system and includes the functionality of the Central Contractor Registry (CCR), Federal Agency Registration (Fedreg), Online Representations and Certifications Application, and the Exclusions Extract. SAM is a Federal government site intended to streamline information for providers [53].

It is important to note that an HHS-OIG exclusion does not technically prohibit individuals or entities from participating in Federal programs, but it does prohibit them from receiving Federal payment for items or services they furnished. "Furnished" is a key word—it refers to items or services provided directly or indirectly by an excluded individual or entity [54].

According to HHS-OIG, "The effect of an OIG exclusion is that no Federal health care program payment may be made for any items or services furnished (1) by an excluded person or (2) at the medical direction or on the prescription of an excluded person" [55]. All claims furnished or submitted by an excluded individual or entity may be considered overpayments subject to recoupment. In addition, the transportation entity may be liable for civil monetary penalties and possible exclusion from Medicaid and other Federal health care program participation. Almost anyone can face exclusion.

CMS has issued guidance to SMAs stating that they should require providers to screen their employees and contractors for exclusions by checking the LEIE database on a monthly basis. The guidance further advises States to require all providers to immediately report any exclusion information discovered. States can find the guidance in State Medicaid Director Letter Number 09-001 [56]. Providers should check the SAM Exclusions Extract as well.

To prevent hiring excluded individuals or entities, implement a process for exclusion screening. It is the business owner's responsibility to make sure they do not employee or contract with excluded individuals. Check for excluded individuals by visiting the LEIE at https://oig.hhs.gov/exclusions/index.asp on the HHS-OIG website and SAM Exclusions Extract at https://www.sam.gov/portal/SAM/#1 on the SAM website. Visit https://oig.hhs.gov/exclusions/tips.asp for quick tips on how to use the HHS-OIG website. The Exclusions FAQ (frequently asked questions) section on the HHS-OIG website has additional information [57].

Report Fraud and Abuse

Report suspected fraud or abuse! Most States do a preliminary investigation and determine whether to send the case to the MFCU. Some States may have regulatory language requiring reporting simultaneously to the SMA and MFCU. Check with your SMA for reporting procedures and document any cases reported to the SMA or MFCU.

- SMA and MFCU https://www.cms.gov/medicare-medicaid-coordination/ fraud-prevention/fraudabuseforconsumers/report_fraud_and_ suspected_fraud.html
- HHS-OIG
  ATTN: Hotline
  P.O. Box 23489
  Washington, DC 20026

Phone: 1-800-447-8477 (1-800-HHS-TIPS)
TTY: 1-800-377-4950
Fax: 1-800-223-8164
Email: HHSTips@oig.hhs.gov
Website: https://forms.oig.hhs.gov/hotlineoperations/

CONCLUSION

Fraud and abuse carry consequences for perpetrators. Penalties depend on the act and the intent. Those found guilty might have to repay Medicaid funds and pay fines and penalties; might be excluded from Federal programs; or might face probation, house arrest, or prison. Medicaid fraud and abuse are serious offenses; be part of the solution.

Medicaid NEMT is an important and necessary service for beneficiaries who do not have the means to get to and from their medical appointments. Everyone associated with Medicaid transportation must play their part to stop fraud and abuse. Be aware of the rules pertaining to each State Medicaid program where services are furnished. Be sure to document furnished services and that the documentation is accurate and complete by verifying services occurred as recorded. Then bill them correctly and be sure there are no excluded individuals or entities on staff. Following the rules of Medicaid and these tips will protect the Medicaid transportation program along with the provider, the provider's employees, and the beneficiaries.

To see the electronic version of this booklet and the other products included in the "Non-Emergency Medical Transportation" Toolkit, visit the Medicaid Program Integrity Education page at https://www.cms.gov/Medicare-Medicaid-Coordination/Fraud-Prevention/Medicaid-Integrity-Education/edmic-landing.html on the CMS website.

REFERENCES

[1] Assurance of Transportation, 42 C.F.R. § 431.53. Retrieved March 15, 2016, from http://www.ecfr.gov/cgibin/retrieveECFR?gp=&SID=0c7ee7a5cbe463eda67e0e61810a8627&mc=true&n=pt42.4.431&r=PART&ty=H TML#se42.4.431_153.

[2] Definitions and Use of Terms, 42 C.F.R. § 435.4. Beneficiary. Retrieved March 15, 2016, from http://www.ecfr. gov/cgi-bin/text-idx?SID=f3a933445ef67278bd2f009091b1703a&mc=true&node=se42.4.435_14&rgn=div8.

[3] Social Security Act § 1902(a)(30)(A). Retrieved March 15, 2016, from https://www.ssa.gov/OP_Home/ssact/ title19/1902.htm.

[4] Sufficiency of Amount, Duration, and Scope, 42 C.F.R. § 440.230. Retrieved March 15, 2016, from http://www. ecfr.gov/cgi-bin/retrieveECFR?gp=&SID=8d4b1988f423f6b72dd99cb4b9ef250a&mc=true&n=pt42.4.440&r=P ART&ty=HTML#se42.4.440_1230.

[5] Covered Services. (2014, June 7). 471 Neb. Admin. Code § 27-002. Retrieved March 15, 2016, from http://www. sos.ne.gov/rules-and-regs/regsearch/Rules/Health_and_Human_Services_System/Title-471/Chapter-27.pdf

[6] Social Security Act § 1932(b)(2)(C). Emergency Medical Condition Defined. Retrieved March 15, 2016, from https://www.ssa.gov/OP_Home/ssact/title19/1932.htm.

[7] Social Security Act § 1902(a)(70). Retrieved March 15, 2016, from https://www.ssa.gov/OP_Home/ssact/ title19/1902.htm.

[8] Assurance of Transportation, 42 C.F.R. § 431.53. Retrieved March 15, 2016, from http://www.ecfr.gov/cgibin/retrieveECFR?gp=&SID=0c7ee7a5cbe463eda67e0e61810a8627&mc=true&n=pt42.4.431&r=PART&ty=H TML#se42.4.431_153.

[9] Social Security Act § 1902(a)(70). Retrieved March 15, 2016, from https://www.ssa.gov/OP_Home/ssact/title19/1902.htm.

[10] Any Other Medical Care or Remedial Care Recognized Under State Law and Specified by the Secretary, 42 C.F.R. 440.170(a)(1). Retrieved March 15, 2016, from http://www.ecfr.gov/cgi-bin/retrieveECFR?gp=&SID=8d4b1988f423f6b72dd99cb4b9ef250a&mc=true&n=pt42.4.440&r=PART&ty=HTML#se42.4.440_1170

[11] Government Accountability Office. (2016, February). Nonemergency Medical Transportation: Updated Medicaid Guidance Could Help States (pp. 8–9). Retrieved March 15, 2016, from http://www.gao.gov/assets/680/674934.pdf.

[12] Any Other Medical Care or Remedial Care Recognized Under State Law and Specified by the Secretary, 42 C.F.R. § 440.170(a)(4) and (a)(4)(i). Retrieved March 15, 2016, from http://www.ecfr.gov/cgi-bin/retrieveECFR?gp=&SID=8d4b1988f423f6b72dd99cb4b9ef250a&mc=true&n=pt42.4.440&r=PART&ty=HTML# se42.4.440_1170.

[13] Education Advisory Committee. Conference Call. (2013, January 30).
[14] Service Definitions: Loaded Mileage. (2014, July 23). 471 Neb. Admin. Code § 27-001. Retrieved March 15, 2016, from http://www.sos.ne.gov/rules-and-regs/regsearch/Rules/Health_and_Human_Services_System/Title-471/Chapter-27.pdf.
[15] False, Fictitious, or Fraudulent Claims, 18 U.S.C. § 287. Retrieved March 15, 2016, from https://www.gpo. gov/fdsys/pkg/USCODE-2011-title18/pdf/USCODE-2011-title18-partI-chap15-sec287.pdf.
[16] Department of Health. New York State Medicaid Program. (2014, September 15). Transportation Manual Policy Guidelines (pp. 30–31; 39; 46–47). Retrieved March 15, 2016, from https://www.emedny.org/ProviderManuals/Transportation/PDFS/Transportation_Manual_Policy_Section.pdf.
[17] Education Advisory Committee. Conference Call. (2013, January 30).
[18] Any Other Medical Care or Remedial Care Recognized Under State Law and Specified by the Secretary, 42 C.F.R. § 440.170(a)(4). Retrieved March 15, 2016, from http://www.ecfr.gov/cgi-bin/retrieveECFR?gp=&SID=8d4b1988f423f6b72dd99cb4b9ef250a&mc=true&n=pt42.4.440&r=PART&ty=HTML#se42.4.440_1170.
[19] Social Security Act § 1902(a)(70)(B)(i). Retrieved March 15, 2016, from https://www.ssa.gov/OP_Home/ ssact/title19/1902.htm
[20] Social Security Act § 1902(a)(70)(B)(ii). Retrieved March 15, 2016, from https://www.ssa.gov/OP_Home/ ssact/title19/1902.htm.
[21] Driver Qualifications. (2014, July 23). 471 Neb. Admin. Code § 27-007.05. Retrieved March 15, 2016, from http://www.sos.ne.gov/rules-and-regs/regsearch/Rules/Health_and_Human_Services_System/Title-471/ Chapter-27.pdf.
[22] Non-Emergency Medical Transportation Service. (2011, September 29). Ohio Admin. Code. § 173-39-02.13 (C)(4)(a)(ii). Retrieved March 15, 2016, from http://codes.ohio.gov/oac/173-39-02.13.
[23] Utah Medicaid Provider Manual. Division of Medicaid and Health Financing, (2015, July). Medical Transportation (§ 1-1, p. 3). Retrieved March 15, 2016, from https://medicaid.utah.gov/Documents/manuals/pdfs/Medicaid%20Provider%20Manuals/Medical%20Transportation/Trans7-15.pdf.
[24] U.S. Department of Health and Human Services. Office of Inspector General. (2014, October). Texas Did Not Always Comply With Federal and State Requirements for Claims Submitted for the Nonemergency

Medical Transportation Program (pp. 5–6). Retrieved March 15, 2016, from https://oig.hhs.gov/oas/reports/region6/61200053.pdf.

[25] U.S. Department of Health and Human Services. Office of Inspector General. (2014, October). Texas Did Not Always Comply With Federal and State Requirements for Claims Submitted for the Nonemergency Medical Transportation Program (pp. 5–6). Retrieved March 15, 2016, from https://oig.hhs.gov/oas/reports/region6/61200053.pdf.

[26] State of Minnesota. Office of the Legislative Auditor. Program Evaluation Division. (2011, February). Evaluation Report: Medical Nonemergency Transportation (p. 62). Retrieved March 15, 2016, from http://www. auditor.leg.state.mn.us/ped/pedrep/mnet.pdf.

[27] South Carolina Department of Health and Human Services. Transportation Advisory Committee. (2014, June 26). Retrieved March 15, 2016, from https://www.scdhhs.gov/meeting-announcement/transportation-advisorycommittee-62614.

[28] State of Wisconsin. Legislative Audit Bureau. (2015, May). Non-Emergency Medical Transportation: Department of Health Services (pp. 43–57). Retrieved March 15, 2016, from http://legis.wisconsin.gov/lab/reports/15-4full.pdf.

[29] Illinois Department of Healthcare and Family Services. (2008, August). Handbook for Providers of Transportation Services §§ T-201.1 Participation Requirements; T-205 Record Requirements. Retrieved March 15, 2016, from http://www.hfs.illinois.gov/assets/t200.pdf.

[30] Department of Health. New York State Medicaid Program. (2014, September 15). Transportation Manual Policy Guidelines (pp. 5, 7, 29–31, 58). Retrieved March 15, 2016, from https://www.emedny.org/ProviderManuals/Transportation/PDFS/Transportation_Manual_Policy_Section.pdf.

[31] Education Advisory Committee. Conference Call. (2013, January 30).

[32] U.S. Department of Health and Human Services. Office of Inspector General. (2015, January). California Claimed Medicaid Reimbursement for Some Nonemergency Medical Transportation Services That Did Not Comply With Federal and State Requirements. Retrieved March 15, 2016, from http://oig.hhs.gov/oas/reports/region9/91302033.pdf.

[33] Definitions, 42 C.F.R. § 455.2. Retrieved March 15, 2016, from http://www.ecfr.gov/cgi-bin/text-idx?SID=48e79f50a55bfc4ad7f5d42cc1751540&mc=true&node=se42.4.455_12&rgn=div8.

[34] Definitions, 42 C.F.R. § 455.2. Retrieved March 15, 2016, from http://www.ecfr.gov/cgi-bin/text-idx?SID=48e79f50a55bfc4ad7f5d42c c1751540&mc=true&node=se42.4.455_12&rgn=div8.
[35] State of Idaho. Office of Attorney General. (2012, June 4). Idaho Falls Woman Sentenced for Medicaid Fraud. Retrieved March 15, 2016, from http://www.ag.idaho.gov/media/newsReleases/2012/nr_06042012.html.
[36] U.S. Attorney's Office. Eastern District of Pennsylvania. (2015, March 10). Medicare Beneficiary Pleads Guilty To Receiving Kickbacks In Health Care Matters. Retrieved April 6, 2016, from https://www. justice.gov/ usao-edpa/pr/medicare-beneficiary-pleads-guilty-receiving-kickbacks-health-care-matters.
[37] U.S. Attorney's Office. Northern District of Indiana. (2015, December 4). Wanda C. Shorter Found Guilty by Jury Trial. Retrieved April 6, 2016, from https://www.justice.gov/usao-ndin/pr/wanda-c-shorter-found-guiltyjury-trial.
[38] Wisconsin Department of Justice. Office of Attorney General. (2012, May 1). Milwaukee Company Convicted of Medicaid Fraud. Retrieved March 15, 2016, from https://www.doj.state.wi.us/news-releases/milwa ukeecompany-convicted-medicaid-fraud.
[39] Branch, A. (2015, September 9). Westchester Man Sentenced in $200,000 Medicaid Fraud. Tarrytown-Sleepy Hollow Patch. Retrieved April 6, 2016, from http://patch.com/new-york/tarrytown/westchester-man-sentenced200000-medicaid-fraud.
[40] New York State. Office of Attorney General. (2015, May 6). A.G. Schneiderman Announces Guilty Plea and Jail Sentence for Owner of Westchester Transportation Company Who Stole More Than $200,000 From Medicaid. Retrieved April 6, 2016, from http://www.ag.ny.gov/ press-release/ag-schneiderman-announces-guiltyplea-and-jail-sentence-owner-westchester.
[41] State of Alaska Department of Law. (2012, December 18). Anchorage Taxi Driver Convicted for Fraudulently Billing Medicaid. Retrieved March 15, 2016, from http://www.law.state.ak.us/press/releases/ 2012/121812- MFCU-Gunes.html.
[42] Social Security Act § 1902(a)(27). Retrieved March 15, 2016, from https://www.ssa.gov/OP_Home/ssact/title19/1902.htm.
[43] Louisiana Medicaid Program. (2014, January 31). Medical Transportation Provider Manual, § 10.6 NEMT—Record Keeping (p. 1 of 2). Retrieved March 15, 2016, from http://www.lamedicaid.

com/provweb1/Providermanuals/manuals/MED_TRANS/MED_TRANS.pdf.

[44] Education Advisory Committee. Conference Call. (2013, January 30).

[45] Education Advisory Committee. Conference Call. (2013, January 30).

[46] Department of Health. New York State Medicaid Program. (2015, September 15). Transportation Manual Policy Guidelines (pp. 7–8). Retrieved March 15, 2016, from https://www.emedny.org/ProviderManuals/Transportation/PDFS/Transportation_Manual_Policy_Section.pdf.

[47] Centers for Medicare & Medicaid Services. CMS-1500 Claim Form (p. 2). Retrieved March 15, 2016, from https://www.cms.gov/Medicare/CMS-Forms/CMS-Forms/Downloads/C MS1500805.pdf.

[48] Centers for Medicare & Medicaid Services. (2006, October). Reference Guide for Medicare Physician & Supplier Billers. Second Edition (pp. 48–49). Retrieved March 15, 2016, from http://amcp.org/WorkArea/DownloadAsset.aspx?id=11778.

[49] Centers for Medicare & Medicaid Services. (2009, January 16). State Medicaid Director Letter 09-001. Policy Clarification: States Should Advise Medicaid Providers to Screen for Exclusions (p. 4). Retrieved April 6, 2016, from https://downloads.cms.gov/cmsgov/archived-downloads/SMDL/downloads/SMD011609.pdf.

[50] System for Award Management. Home Page. Retrieved March 15, 2016, from https://www.sam.gov/portal/SAM/#1.

[51] Social Security Act § 1128. Exclusion of Certain Individuals and Entities From Participation in Medicare and State Health Care Programs. Retrieved March 15, 2016, from https://www.ssa.gov/OP_Home/ssact/title11/ 1128.htm.

[52] U.S. Department of Health and Human Services. Office of Inspector General. List of Excluded Individuals and Entities. Retrieved March 15, 2016, from https://oig.hhs.gov/exclusions/index.asp.

[53] System for Award Management. General Information. Retrieved March 15, 2016, from https://www.sam.gov/ portal/SAM/#1.

[54] Scope and Effect of Exclusion, 42 C.F.R. § 1001.1901(b)(1). Retrieved March 15, 2016, from http://www. ecfr.gov/cgi-bin/text-idx?SID=1016abaf96aa817ab318a1da01d73f4c&mc=true&node=se42.5.1001_11901& rgn=div8.

[55] U.S. Department of Health and Human Services. Office of Inspector General. (2013, May 8). Special Advisory Bulletin on the Effect of Exclusion from Participation in Federal Health Care Programs: Updated.

Retrieved March 15, 2016, from https://oig.hhs.gov/exclusions/files/sab-05092013.pdf.

[56] Centers for Medicare & Medicaid Services. (2009, January 16). State Medicaid Director Letter 09-001. Policy Clarification: States Should Advise Medicaid Providers to Screen for Exclusions (p. 4). Retrieved April 6, 2016, from https://downloads.cms.gov/cmsgov/archived-downloads/SMDL/downloads/SMD011609.pdf.

[57] U.S. Department of Health and Human Services. Office of Inspector General. Exclusions FAQ. Retrieved March 15, 2016, from https://oig.hhs.gov/faqs/exclusions-faq.asp.

RELATED NOVA PUBLICATION

TRANSPORTATION SERVICES FOR OLDER ADULTS AND NONEMERGENCY MEDICAL TRANSPORTATION: SELECTED ANALYSES

Patricia Harris-Bowen

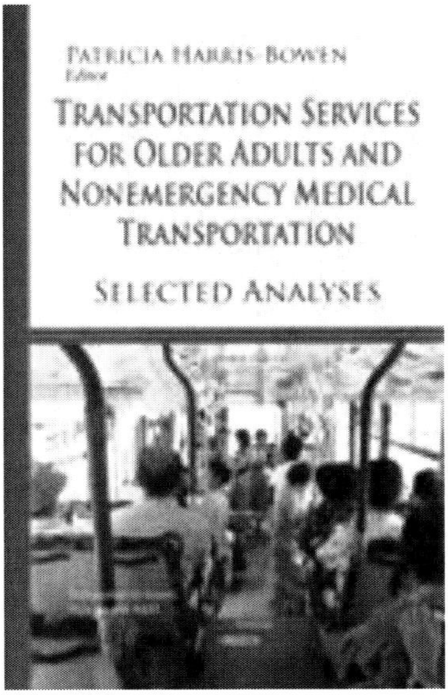

ISBN: 978-1-63482-569-6 Publication Date: 2015

As the U.S. population ages, access to safe and reliable transportation alternatives is critical to helping older adults remain in their homes as long as possible. HHS, DOT, VA, and other federal agencies may provide funds to state and local entities to help older adults access transportation. This book examines the federal programs that provide funding for transportation services for older adults and the extent to which the programs that fund these services are coordinated; and how state and local transportation agencies and aging network organizations in selected states coordinate transportation for older adults and the challenges they face in coordinating or providing these services. The book also addresses the federal programs that provide funding for NEMT services; how federal agencies are coordinating NEMT services; and how NEMT services are coordinated at the state and local levels and the challenges to coordination.

INDEX

I

L

M

N

O

P

U

V

W